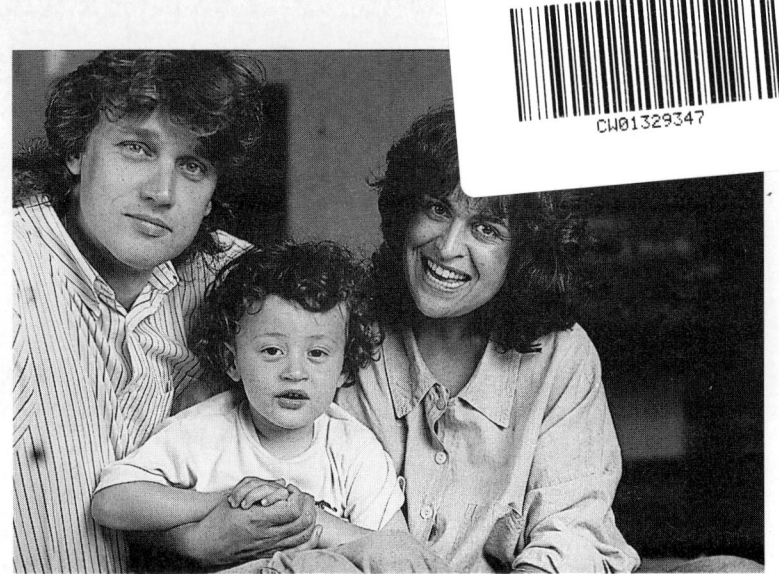

Photo: Jane Bown

Anna Knopfler developed diabetes at the age of 27 while working as a teacher in London. Her son Jackson was born in August 1985. It was during her pregnancy that she discovered how limited information on pregnancy and diabetes was for women like herself. This prompted her to form the Diabetic Pregnancy Network, an organisation to put pregnant diabetic women in touch with each other. Anna is married to composer and musician David Knopfler.

OPTIMA

DIABETES AND PREGNANCY

ANNA KNOPFLER

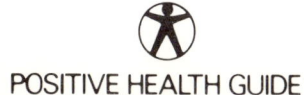

POSITIVE HEALTH GUIDE

© Anna Knopfler 1989

First published in 1989 by
Macdonald Optima, a division of
Macdonald & Co. (Publishers) Ltd

A member of Maxwell Pergamon Publishing Corporation plc

All rights reserved

No part of this publication may be reproduced,
stored in a retrieval system, or transmitted,
in any form or by any means without the prior
permission in writing of the publisher, nor be
otherwise circulated in any form of binding or
cover other than that in which it is published
and without a similar condition including this
condition being imposed on the subsequent
purchaser.

British Library Cataloguing in Publication Data
Knopfler, Anna
   Diabetes and pregnancy.
   1. Pregnant women. Diabetes
   I. Title   II. Series
   618.3

   ISBN 0-356-15189-1

Macdonald & Co. (Publishers) Ltd
66–73 Shoe Lane
London EC4P 4AB

Photoset in 11pt Times by Tek Art Limited, Croydon, Surrey

Printed in Great Britain at the University Press, Cambridge

CONTENTS

	Foreword	vi
	Preface	vii
	Acknowledgments	viii
1	Introduction	1
2	Pre-conception	6
3	Antenatal care	19
4	Maintaining balance	35
5	Gestational diabetes	51
6	Keeping healthy	57
7	Nutrition and pregnancy	72
8	Labour	83
9	Breastfeeding	102
10	The baby	116
11	Managing the baby and your diabetes	125
12	Sex and contraception	133
13	Quick questions and answers	143
	Glossary	147
	Useful addresses and telephone numbers	155
	Index	166

FOREWORD

Anna Knopfler has diabetes. After her pregnancy, acting on her own experience and that of other diabetic women, she has written a comprehensive book about diabetes and pregnancy. She stresses that the diabetic who understands her illness, takes control of it and who is motivated to seek pre-conceptual advice has an excellent chance of having a relatively uncomplicated pregnancy and confinement. Anna has included a chapter of answers to common queries, a glossary defining medical terms and an extensive list of useful addresses and telephone numbers to which a diabetic woman may easily refer for further information. Anna has succeeded in her aims to inform and enlighten diabetic women.

I thoroughly recommend this book.

Moira Kelly, FRCOG
Norwich, 1988

PREFACE

Some time after the birth of our son, I wrote to *Balance*, the magazine published by the British Diabetic Association, asking women to write to me about their experiences of pregnancy and diabetes. I wanted to set up an organisation where women could talk to each other about their pregnancy, and I also felt there was a pressing need for information. Over 100 women wrote to me describing, often in great detail, the events surrounding the birth of their children. They certainly made interesting reading and often put me in mind of the comment made to me by a diabetic physician: 'The treatment you receive depends on the doctor you get!' Opinions and practices seem to vary enormously; the points made by women ranged from 'I have every confidence in my doctor' to 'I was frightened and very humiliated by the way I had been treated.'

Certain doctors, hospitals and clinics were praised over and over again by their patients. Unfortunately, though, a great number of letters catalogued a wide variety of complaints. They generally fell into three clear categories.

- Lack of information. This was the most frequently mentioned. In fact there are a number of salutary articles on the subject of pregnancy and diabetes, but it is up to the reader to hunt them out. The British Diabetic Association has now prepared a pregnancy pack, available on request, in order to rectify this situation.
- Seemingly unnecessary and unexplained inductions and caesarean sections. All the women who wrote to me were bright people who knew a great deal about pregnancy, and would have appreciated more dialogue on these subjects.

- Not being believed or treated as an intelligent adult. Complaints of this nature were often horrendous. More compassion please!

I hope this book will answer all the questions you may have, as well as provide a sufficient amount of information to enable you to choose certain aspects of your baby's birth. It is written from the patient's point of view and certainly answers all my own queries. Let's hope it will go some way towards ensuring that we diabetic women all have healthy happy babies and a trouble-free nine months.

ACKNOWLEDGMENTS

I would like to thank all the women (and those few men) who took the time to write to me. I would also like to express my gratitude to the staff at Queen Charlotte's Maternity Hospital in London where Jackson was delivered. Thanks also to all the doctors who answered my questions and kept me well; to Suzanne Redmond who graciously assisted me in my research; and to Harriet Griffey, the editor whose judgment proved invaluable. Many thanks to Jane Bown and Gavin Cochrane for their photographs. Finally, thank you Becton Dickinson for paying my secretarial costs.

Special thanks and love to my husband David who supported the writing of this book in innumerable ways.

The publishers would like to thank AMT Advanced Medical Technology, Cambridge; Chefaro Proprietaries Ltd, Science Park, Cambridge; Department of Medical Illustration, John Radcliffe Hospital, Oxford; Diabetic Care Ltd/Norman Mays Studio; Sally and Richard Greenhill; Daisy Hays; Dr R. Holman, Diabetes Research Laboratories, Radcliffe Infirmary, Oxford; Hypoguard (UK) Ltd, Camilla Jessel; Jenny Matthews/Format; Medic-Alert Foundation; Science Photo Library; the Whittington Hospital; and Zefa for the photographs; and Maggie Raynor for the line illustrations.

1

INTRODUCTION

The following account will give you some idea of the processes normally involved in having diabetes and being pregnant.

I am an insulin-dependent diabetic with a three-month-old baby boy, Michael David. Diabetes is a chronic disorder affecting the secretion of insulin (the hormone which makes it possible for the body to utilise sugar) from the pancreas. In the undiagnosed diabetic the sugar accumulates in the blood with distressing effects on the person; they become thirsty, tired and unwell and it is essential that they receive medical treatment promptly. Most diabetics of child-bearing age require insulin which is administered by injection twice daily. Failure to eat at regular times can cause low blood sugar. A high-fibre carbohydrate-controlled diet and regular meals are essential for good control. In order to maintain good control diabetics measure their blood-sugar levels, and in pregnancy this can mean up to seven times daily. Blood-sugar levels must be kept as near to normal as possible as there could be a harmful effect on the fetus. I used a Glucochek meter to record my own blood-sugar levels.

My GP booked me into hospital on 19 February when I attended the Tuesday morning diabetic antenatal clinic. The clinic checks diabetic control, blood pressure and heart, as well as doing routine obstetric checks. My insulin was changed to a mixture of cloudy (Insulatard) and clear (Velosulin) insulin. My daily dose was increased to maintain good control. (I had previously taken 36 units a day of Mixtard insulin.)

On 3 April I had my first scan and an alphafetoprotein check for spina bifida (fortunately all was well). On 20 April I first felt 'Junior' moving, whilst listening to a concert. I had a scan at each subsequent visit to the clinic (every four weeks at this stage). By the end of May my insulin requirements had greatly increased. On 11 June I attended hospital for a fetal heart scan – very illuminating. I know more about the inside than the outside of my baby.

I was admitted to the hospital ward on 1 September and was to be induced at 38 weeks the following day. Junior's weight was then over 8 lb (3.6 kg). Diabetics always used to be induced early as there is a greater risk of toxaemia, but now many are allowed to go full term. I had high blood pressure. On 2 September I was taken to the labour ward with my husband Graham, and they started to induce me at 9.15 am with pessaries. The baby was monitored throughout. My waters were broken at 2 pm. I was 'taped down' to the bed with an insulin/glucose drip to maintain good diabetic control and to feed me, and I was also attached to a hormone drip to encourage the uterus to contract – which it did later, very violently! I was taken to the delivery room at 8 pm and awaited my epidural, which was administered at 11 pm. By now my contractions were very intense, and Graham was a great support, despite having his hair pulled out. I was given pethidine, which made me feel woozy. It was so blissful after the epidural – now no pain! However, the baby had suffered and they decided to deliver me right away by emergency caesarean under epidural. Michael David arrived in the world at 00.28 am on 3 September weighing 8 lb 10½ oz (3.9 kg). I felt very sleepy, my insulin/glucose drip and catheter were removed the following day, and I returned to my ward. Michael David was taken into special care as he had low blood sugar. The normal ward routine for diabetics includes checking urine four times daily for protein, ketones, blood and sugar and also checking blood-sugar levels. I was returned to my pre-pregnancy insulin on 4 September.

Michael David was breastfed, but he seemed fractious and difficult to settle. He was also jaundiced. I was discharged from hospital after a week and then readjusted to my new lifestyle, which did take me some time. Michael David is now 12 weeks old and is progressing well.   *Tina*

I believe that most people, when told they are suffering from diabetes, go through the same separate stages of acknowledging the disease and thereafter coping with it. Certainly, speaking for myself, it took me a great deal of time to accept my condition. For the initial six months following diagnosis I suffered from depression. The diabetes, in itself, was not giving me any problems. My diet and insulin dosage were well controlled; I followed all the advice I had been given by both doctors and dietitians and was classified as reasonably stable; I could handle the counting out of carbohydrate portions and, although I occasionally misjudged a meal, there were no serious mistakes. My depression resulted not from these things, but from the idea and routine of the diabetic condition – a lifetime's concentration of energy to be expended every breakfast, lunch and dinner. I felt suddenly imprisoned and unable to explain the daily complications. People generally surmise that, once insulin has been prescribed for the sufferer and the insulin is taken regularly, then the problem subsides. But this is often not the case.

It took me quite some time to emerge from these intense feelings of restriction to those approaching relative normality. However, although I felt less insecure and vulnerable, I still was not dealing with the fact that I had diabetes. I rarely admitted to people that I suffered from the disease. I made no allowances whatsoever for it, continuing to smoke and occasionally to drink to excess. I rarely tested my blood glucose. At that time the most acceptable and cheapest method of testing was by urine sample. Later, when glucose test strips were issued, they remained unused in a drawer. The only times I became concerned about test results were when a visit to the clinic loomed. I became anxious and unhappy for a whole week preceding my appointment. In fact the months leading up to a clinic visit were akin to walking slowly towards a firing range. This stage lasted some years and frequently other people had to pick up the pieces.

My clinic visits at this time consisted of no more than a five-minute consultation with a junior doctor I had never seen before and was unlikely to see again. I knew that my medical notes had not been looked at. There simply wasn't the time or money for an efficient service. Another 30 people were waiting in line behind me. After at least an hour and a half's wait I was treated as a 'stupid woman', or as someone who needed the basics of diabetes explaining yet again, or as another number in a busy afternoon, or as a reasonably intelligent human being whom the doctor didn't have time to talk to intelligently. After each visit I went straight to the hospital shop and bought a large bar of chocolate as a reward for having done it! I'm sure diabetic clinics have changed a lot since I last attended one in 1983 – although I'm equally sure a number haven't.

I had had diabetes for about six years before the night when I was found in a deep coma by my husband. It took several hours for the hospital to bring me round. This was the first, and hopefully the last, time I've experienced a hypoglycaemic coma. It took a couple of weeks to restabilise me and I was then discharged fit and well. It was after this episode that I moved onto the final stage of dealing with the disease.

Having frightened my husband considerably, I promised him I would not go to sleep without testing my blood glucose again. From this point in my life I decided to take full charge. I realised it simply wasn't fair on other people to expect them to cope with a disease I was constantly dismissing, and since then I have never missed a day without testing. I feel remarkably well, both physically and mentally, and I find the diabetes easier to accept now that I dominate it, instead of it dominating me. Thankfully I had taken this momentous decision before I conceived.

I became pregnant at the age of 35, very soon after discontinuing contraception. At the time I was taking one insulin injection in the morning. At approximately six weeks' gestation I privately visited a diabetes consultant who carefully spelled out the importance of good control during the nine-month period and immediately switched me to two injections a day, which would help facilitate near normal blood-glucose levels. He also made me aware of pre-conception counselling.

At this point I hunted around for information on the subject. It took quite some searching to get all the details that I wanted, and the results of this research had a somewhat chilling effect. The material shouted about stillbirths, congenital defects and emergency caesareans. This frightened me, as I was not perfectly controlled in the first few weeks of pregnancy, although I was for the rest of the seven-and-a-half months.

At the time I conceived I wasn't smoking or drinking. I was exercising on a bike for 20 minutes a day. I wasn't eating meat at all, but plenty of fish, nuts and pulses. My diet was low in fats and was absent in tea and coffee. I also took one multivitamin tablet a day and two vitamin B_{12} tablets, which I continued to take during pregnancy. My husband was also fit and well.

At no time during gestation did I experience any problems. Altogether I had four ultrasound scans which showed the healthy normal development of the baby, much to my relief, and all the other tests I had showed that everything was fine. My blood-glucose readings remained within the normal range at all times. In fact in the last two months I kept the levels slightly lower than 5 mmol, as I was advised to do so.

The one thing I wanted to avoid was a caesarean section. I hoped to have a natural birth, but chose eventually to have an epidural. A few days before my due date I went into labour at home and we drove to the hospital. I spent a few hours without drugs, moving around freely. My blood sugar was 6 mmol and was tested at regular intervals. I then asked for an epidural, which was duly administered. My readings remained at 6 mmol throughout labour, without recourse to insulin and glucose drips.

Our son was eventually born at the end of an 11½-hour labour, delivered normally and weighing a healthy 8 pounds (3.6 kg). He did not need the services of special care and I was able to feed him on the delivery table. I felt utterly triumphant with joy.

I have now had diabetes for 11 years and manage the disease easily using an insulin pen. I find I have the same sense of freedom that a non-diabetic enjoys: I no longer have to stop what I'm doing when it's 12 o'clock; I no longer have to eat when I'm not hungry. I reached this happy plateau, however, only after a great deal of wretchedness. Surely some form of routine qualified counselling should co-exist within the diabetic clinic duties. After all, in the end, it is the individual's attitude to her disease which has the most effect on it!

2

PRE-CONCEPTION

All the recent research into pregnancy and diabetes has stressed the need for good pre-conceptual care. Dr Judith M. Steele set up the first diabetic pre-conception clinic of its kind in this country in order to help women with diabetes have successful pregnancies and births. These are her comments on the subject.

All pregnancies should be planned but this is particularly important for an insulin-dependent diabetic. Before a formal visit to a pre-pregnancy clinic, possible future pregnancies should be discussed and expert contraceptive advice obtained. The pre-pregnancy clinic itself will usually be run by a diabetic physician, a dietitian and an obstetrician who looks after pregnant diabetics. A formal visit to this clinic is best arranged a few months before a pregnancy is planned and ideally the diabetic and her partner should attend. There are several purposes of a pre-pregnancy clinic, the first being to assess the diabetic's suitability for pregnancy. Fortunately the vast majority of diabetics can and do become pregnant and have normal healthy babies. In a long-standing diabetic it is wise to measure kidney function, to pay particular attention to blood pressure and to carry out an exercise electrocardiogram (ECG). Very rarely, someone with serious complications may be best advised not to become pregnant. Retinopathy is no longer a contraindication to pregnancy but may need treatment before conception. The second purpose is to explain to a prospective mother and her partner exactly what is involved in antenatal care and delivery and why tight control is essential. How to cope with hypoglycaemia, should it be a problem, must also be discussed. Most people will try extremely hard to control their diabetes and keep all their appointments if they know why they are being asked to do this. The third and perhaps most important purpose of a pre-pregnancy clinic is to obtain really good diabetic control at the time of conception. There is a high incidence of congenital abnormalities in infants of diabetic mothers and it has been shown clearly that this is related to control in early pregnancy when the baby is forming (which is at only 6–8 weeks' gestation). The higher the HbA_1 the higher the risk and with really good control the risk seems to be very little if at all above the level in the general population. The fourth purpose is to ensure that mothers present early in pregnancy for antenatal care and that the 'dates' are confirmed by an early scan. Sending off a pregnancy test six weeks after a period and, if it is negative, repeating it until bleeding occurs or it becomes positive ensures very early antenatal care. Also at the clinic any gynaecological problems or previous obstetric problems can be discussed and questions can be answered. German measles immunity is checked and immunisation offered to anyone not already immune. The diet is reviewed and anyone overweight is encouraged to lose weight before conception. Anyone who smokes is very strongly advised to stop. The number of follow-up visits to the pre-pregnancy clinic will depend on how quickly good control can be achieved and any other problems sorted out.

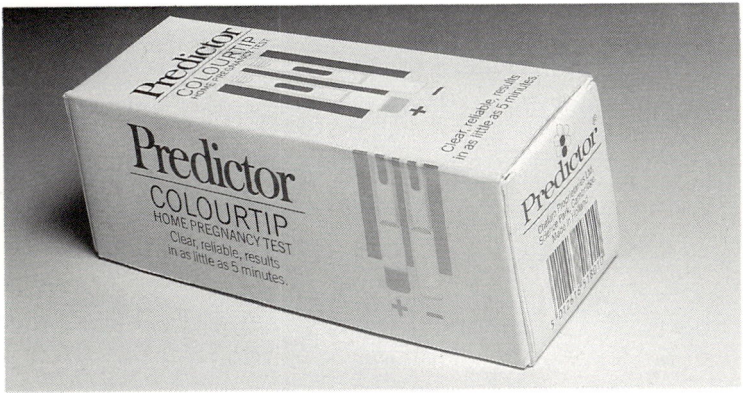

Pregnancy testing kit.

GLYCOSYLATED HAEMOGLOBIN

This test, abbreviated to HbA_1 and mentioned above by Judith Steele, is done simply and regularly throughout a diabetic pregnancy. A small sample of blood is taken from the arm and sent to the laboratory to be analysed. In a non-diabetic person the HbA_1 will be between 5–8.5 mmol. This reading is the one we should all aim for during pregnancy. The test should reassure both patient and doctor alike that good glucose levels have been established and maintained. It will also provide validation for the doctor that testing done at home is accurate.

A DIABETIC PRE-CONCEPTION CLINIC

Many diabetic pre-conception clinics now exist to prepare insulin-dependent women for pregnancy. The following outline of how such a clinic operates may be slightly different from the way another clinic works, but it should give you some idea of what to expect should you be given the opportunity to attend one. Sadly, not all diabetic clinics have pre-conception sessions available.

The department has two consulting rooms, one in the diabetic clinic and one in the maternity hospital. Counselling takes place for between one and six hours per week, once or twice a month. Mothers-to-be are initially seen with their partners at the diabetic clinic. The second session takes place in the obstetric department with the consultant obstetrician and diabetic physician. The mum is subsequently seen as often as is required, in order to maintain good diabetic control – this can involve anything from two to 20 visits.

First visit

At this visit an overall look into the diabetes and general health takes place. Diabetic control is assessed, the eyes are examined, blood pressure is checked and an ECG (to check heart function) may be performed if the diabetes is long standing (over 10 years' duration). The diet is examined and may be revised. Smoking and drinking are discouraged. Pregnancy protocol is discussed and any questions are answered.

Subsequent visits

On the second visit a closer look is taken at the pregnancy, and gynaecological problems are discussed with the obstetrician. On the third visit the HbA$_1$ levels are monitored, and advice is given to the partner on signs of hypoglycaemia and instruction is given on the use of glucagon. Information is also given about pregnancy tests. Further visits will then take place to check progress.

Ignoring the importance of pre-conceptual care can have disastrous results, as this account illustrates.

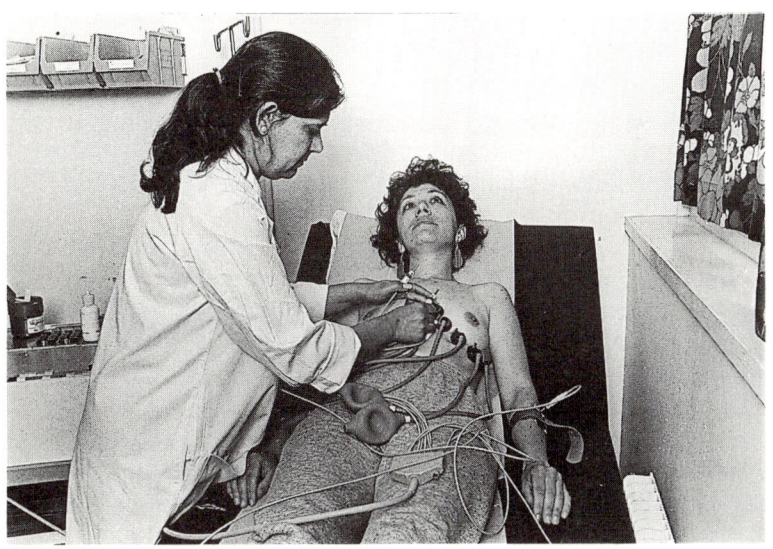

ECG being performed.

I am a 24-year-old insulin-dependent diabetic. I was first diagnosed at the age of seven. Like the majority of diabetics, I neglected my diabetes through adolescence and when I married at the age of 18 I had got to the point where I wasn't seeing a diabetic specialist, only my GP.

Blood-sugar tests and urine tests were non-existent in my regime, and to my knowledge a diabetic pregnancy was no different to any other pregnancy. Unfortunately a visit to my GP before we tried to conceive didn't enlighten me in the least.

I fell pregnant within two months of trying and returned

to my GP immediately. He was most surprised at my ability to conceive and calmly told me to come back in six weeks, for my 12-week appointment at the clinic, and after this I was seen by him at fortnightly intervals – still none the wiser, and still no mention of any blood sugars.

Finally at 18 weeks of pregnancy I was referred to a consultant obstetrician and immediately admitted into hospital for a blood-sugar profile and scan. My minimum reading was 17 mmol. My insulin dosage was readjusted and my blood sugars seemed to level out. However, I spent many more weeks in hospital throughout my pregnancy as I developed oedema, gaining 5½ stone (35 kg) in weight, and my blood sugars continued to be erratic. The swelling became worse and at 34 weeks an amniocentesis was performed which showed the baby's lungs were mature enough to withstand an early delivery.

Our daughter Danielle was delivered by caesarean, weighing a hefty, but rather unhealthy, 8 lb 10 oz (3.9 kg). She developed severe breathing difficulties and was admitted to special care. Much to my distress and objections I was unable to see her until 24 hours later. I had to rely on comments from my husband and the hospital staff as to my daughter's resemblances and loveliness. When I finally saw her I was unable to hold her. She was in an incubator connected to every conceivable tube and drip possible. She was very big for dates, but oh such a beautiful baby.

I was quite concerned about her breathing and expressed this concern to the paediatrician. I was told it was normal for babies of unstable diabetics to have such problems. However, after two days Danielle showed no improvement and the staff carried out further investigations. The result of these showed that Danielle had some problem with her heart. She was transferred to the local children's hospital which had specialised equipment. This showed that Danielle's heart was on the right instead of the left and that her top two chambers were joined together, making a total of three chambers instead of four. The hospital staff felt there were also probably other problems with her heart, but the only way to detect these was by cardiac catheterisation which could cause serious complications in such a young baby. They decided to postpone it until she was older. However, after weeks of constant heart failure Danielle was readmitted to hospital for catheterisation. The results were a horrific blow. As well as Danielle's heart being on the right and the chambers being joined together, she had seven tubes going into the heart instead of six, and instead of them going into the different chambers, they all went into one. The valves on the bottom right-hand chamber hadn't formed properly, making corrective surgery almost impossible. Survival without surgery was nil.

The operation, however, wasn't performed, as complications from the catheterisation occurred and Danielle developed a bowel blockage. Aged eight weeks and two days, our darling brave little girl lost her fight for life.

That was five years ago, and afterwards I made sure I knew everything about diabetes and pregnancy. After Danielle's death I saw genetic counsellors and a diabetic specialist, all of whom suggested, although they couldn't prove it, that Danielle's complications arose from my unstable diabetes.

Eighteen months on, after meticulous diabetic control before and during pregnancy, I gave birth to Natalie Jayne. She was delivered at 38 weeks by elective caesarean. She weighed a perfect 6 lb 14 oz (3.1 kg) and was healthy in every way. The importance of good diabetic control was proof of the pudding to me – there was just no comparison at birth between Danielle and Natalie Jayne. She was perfect in every way.

Whilst expecting Natalie I came across a number of girls who were pregnant and had diabetes. The majority of them gave birth to normal healthy babies, but how some of them managed it God only knows. They would sit there sharing Mars bars, pop and packets of crisps by the dozen. I talked to them until I was blue in the face, but none of it sunk in. Two of them did, however, suffer the consequences of their lack of diabetic management. One gave birth at 36 weeks to an 11 lb (5.0 kg) baby with severe breathing difficulties and other complications; sadly she lived only a few hours. The other had a daughter at 37 weeks with minor abnormalities to her ears, fingers and toes. She weighed a rather unhealthy 10 lb 6 oz (4.7 kg) and now three years later it has been discovered she will be incontinent for the rest of her life.

Just after we lost Danielle, a lady in the clinic asked me

if my diabetes had ever caused me any problems? 'Yes', I replied, 'my ignorance of it caused me to lose the most wanted and precious person in our lives.'

Jackie

Some doctors have experienced difficulties with setting up pre-conception clinics due to a lack of interest from their patients. If your diabetic clinic does not provide pregnancy counselling, it may well be because of this. Let your doctors know you want this facility.

The consultant at my diabetic clinic suggested that I attended a pre-conception clinic, where I was given, in detail, all the problem areas about being diabetic and pregnant. I was made fully aware that I had to be well controlled, and why.

Ellie

The clinic doctor organised pre-pregnancy counselling for me last year when I mentioned that I was considering it. This involved seeing the clinic doctor by appointment (not in the clinic, no waiting) every three weeks or so to discuss my control, etc. Once I suspected pregnancy we went up to see the doctor who monitors all the pregnant diabetics and he was really good. He sees all the pregnant women about every week or ten days, all without waiting and usually at a time to suit me. Every now and again he says 'Two more were born last week – normal healthy births', which is quite encouraging. He is also available by phone at any time and never minds being interrupted.

Daphne

If all insulin-dependent women planned their pregnancies, then all the risks associated with the disease would diminish significantly.

WHAT ARE THE RISKS?

For the baby

- Research work with rats has shown that elevated blood

sugar in early pregnancy often results in a high rate of abnormal fetal development.
- Glucose crosses the placenta, whereas insulin doesn't. If the mother's glucose levels are very high, then the pancreas of the baby has to produce more insulin to cope. These abnormal insulin levels often result in macrosomia (large birth weight) and hypoglycaemia once the baby is born.
- Elevated blood-glucose levels in pregnancy often result in the infant being born with respiratory distress syndrome (poor functioning of the lungs, often associated with immature pre-term babies).
- Several researchers have discovered that there is a certain correlation between high HbA_1 levels in early pregnancy and congenital abnormalities in the baby.

For the mother

- If the diabetes is badly controlled then the mother will feel generally unwell throughout her pregnancy.
- Labour will probably be more difficult if good control has not been achieved previously. The likelihood of a caesarean section will increase.
- The mother is more likely to be induced prematurely as the baby may be too large to be born at term. The fetus becomes unusually bloated as a direct result of continued high glucose levels in the mother.
- The mother will probably have to spend time in hospital during pregnancy.
- There is a higher risk of pre-eclampsia (high blood pressure, protein in urine, retention of fluid), which can be life threatening.

ESTABLISHING GOOD CONTROL

If you read this and are already pregnant, don't panic. Over 90 per cent of diabetic women give birth to healthy babies, and not all of the women have planned their pregnancies. However, the risks are considerably reduced when the diabetes is well controlled prior to conception.

This means the levels of glucose present in the blood must be similar to those of a non-diabetic. Although this may seem an impossibility, in fact it is quite easy to achieve. Most diabetic women are highly motivated during pregnancy and often do as many as four blood tests a day, as well as keeping a watchful eye on all other health matters.

What reading should I aim for?
Blood tests should always be between 5–8 mmol. Slightly lower readings should be aimed for in the last three months.

Am I fit to conceive?
Some women with diabetes and other associated diseases may be considered unfit for pregnancy by their doctors and therefore advised against it. Pregnancy in these cases may worsen an already existing condition. If you suffer from any of the following, talk to your doctor before considering pregnancy.

- Retinopathy
- Serious renal disease
- Heart disease

When should I have children?
If diabetes was contracted by a woman when she was a child, then all the risks associated with the disease are accentuated – the longer she has had diabetes, the greater the risks. It is therefore advisable to have children earlier rather than later in life.

TAKE CHARGE OF YOURSELF

The healthier and happier your pregnancy is, the more secure and confident you will feel when the time comes to give birth.

Give up smoking
If you are contemplating pregnancy you want your baby to be healthy. Smoking reduces the oxygen supply to the baby and has an adverse effect on the blood supply to the uterus. Babies born of women who smoke generally weigh less. Ultrasound scans have shown that fetal breathing patterns are disturbed when the mother smokes a cigarette. Any woman with kidney disease, high blood pressure or pre-eclampsia is putting herself

and her baby at serious risk if she smokes. Even passive smoking – being in a smoke-filled environment – is harmful to you and your baby.

Lung cancer is a direct result of the use of cigarettes, while bronchitis and other chest and lung ailments, as well as heart complaints, are common amongst smokers. And there may well be other harmful effects which have not yet been assessed. For the sake of your health and your baby's, try to stop smoking before conception.

Usually planning a pregnancy motivates the mother-to-be to give up smoking. Talk to your doctor about methods that are available which will help you to stop.

Don't drink

Professor Mathew Kaufman, a world expert on early embryology, has found that alcohol consistently consumed before conception can damage the eggs produced by the female. It is widely known that alcohol increases the risk of infertility, miscarriages and various mental and physical handicaps to the fetus. 'In terms of numbers affected, alcohol may be a vastly bigger problem than thalidomide ever was', says Professor Kaufman; there is no safe level of alcohol – 'a toxic level for one could be one drink, for another it could be half a bottle a day!' The only reasonable action to take is not to drink at all prior to conception and during pregnancy.

Alcohol depletes the body of folic acid if taken in the early weeks of pregnancy. Folic acid, one of the B-complex vitamins, is essential for the healthy development of the baby. Many women in early pregnancy are already deficient in this nutrient and alcohol can easily make the situation worse. Drink has the effect of lowering blood sugar and the diabetic mother-to-be may have difficulty in distinguishing the difference between a hypoglycaemic reaction and a feeling of drunkenness. And alcohol crosses the placenta, so if the mother feels tipsy so does the baby.

Many women find the taste of alcohol repugnant whilst pregnant. Perhaps this is nature's way of guarding the well-being of the baby.

Immunity against German measles

If contracted during pregnancy, rubella (German measles) can cause severe abnormalities to the fetus. Before conceiving you must therefore check whether or not you are immune to German measles. Your doctor will take a blood sample and if the test reveals that you lack immunity then inoculation against rubella should be carried out at least three months before attempting to conceive.

Lose weight if overweight

Now is the time to achieve your ideal weight, as recommended by your doctor and dietitian. This may mean losing weight, before you conceive. Your dietitian will look at your diet sheet and advise you on the best methods. Most will advise the following.

- Cut down on red meat.
- Cut down on saturated fats (including high-fat cheeses).
- Increase the proportion of fibre in your meals.
- Count the calories in an average day's intake of food – try and keep the level down to the limit agreed with your dietitian.
- Take more exercise.

Being overweight at the time of conception puts an extra strain on your hardworking body. You may suffer from fatigue more frequently as a result of being too heavy. Many women, if they are carrying extra weight at the time of conception, feel extremely depressed at the idea of nine months of pregnancy. However, pregnancy is not the time to diet, as it can seriously affect the health of the baby. You should aim to achieve your ideal weight before conception.

MATERNAL AGE

Women over 35 years old and having their first baby are termed elderly primigravida by the medical profession. Although this sounds ominous, it does not mean that a healthy woman, even a diabetic, cannot have a successful birth. I was 35 when I had my son and experienced no problems. I had been diagnosed diabetic at the age of 27 years.

Women of childbearing age who have been diabetic for a period of longer than 10 years may prefer to have their babies at a younger rather than older age. Complications of diabetes are certainly more commonly found where the diabetes is longer-term, say 10 years or more. Age should therefore be considered by the diabetic woman, although it should not preclude the birth of a healthy baby.

INFERTILITY

A woman with diabetes is no less fertile than any other woman, so if a couple find difficulty conceiving, a doctor should be consulted as to the cause. There may be many reasons why infertility occurs; certainly a healthy diet with adequate vitamins can improve the chances of conception for both would-be parents.

Adelle Davis was a dedicated nutritionist, believing that better health would be the natural outcome of a good diet. These are her comments on infertility, taken from her book *Let's Have Healthy Children*:

> Vitamin A deficiencies greatly lower experimental fertility and damage the sperm-producing cells in mice. Mild deficiencies of vitamin E allow fewer sperm to be produced, whereas a severe lack may cause sterility in the male. Conversely, when men have increased their vitamin E intake, the quality of their sperm improves markedly, especially if vitamin A and E are taken together.
>
> Inadequate B vitamins and protein limit sperm motility and the production of both ova and sperm. A lack of the B vitamin pantothenic acid or vitamin B_{12} causes infertility in animals and damages the testicles. And when infertile men have taken B_{12} the sperm count has increased from 3 million sluggish cells to 140 million highly active ones.
>
> Lack of manganese or zinc, both often deficient in our soil, markedly decreases fertility in laboratory and farm animals. Too little manganese can even cause a total absence of sperm. If the diet is adequate, zinc, essential to the fertility of both sexes, is found in larger amounts in the sperm, testicles, and prostate than elsewhere in the male's body.
>
> Many women who are sterile when overweight conceive after reducing their weight on a high-protein diet free from refined sugar.

Conversely, failure to conceive can be caused by eating too little, a fact revealed by studies of undernourished women during World War II. Smoking and drinking reduce the number of live sperm and their motility, and conceptions often occur after these habits have been given up.

Adelle Davis

3

ANTENATAL CARE

CHOOSING WHERE TO GIVE BIRTH

Hopefully your blood sugar will be stabilised and the pregnancy a planned one. However, if your control is generally good and you find out you are pregnant without it being planned, there is no reason why the pregnancy shouldn't progress equally as well.

It is at this point when you may wish to find out more information about the hospitals in your area. You are not obliged to have the baby at the hospital where your diabetic clinic is located, although this may be more convenient in terms of travelling time. Here is a list of things you can do in order to assess your local hospitals.

- Join the National Childbirth Trust (see Useful Addresses, page 160). The organisation welcomes members from every class, race and creed so don't be afraid that it isn't for you. Talk to the women in your local group and ask them their opinions of the surrounding hospitals.
- Talk to your GP. Tell him if you are not happy with the hospital you are most likely to be assigned to and ask him to refer you to another.
- Write or phone the senior nursing officer at the hospitals you are interested in and ask them the questions that most concern you.
- Join the Diabetic Pregnancy Network. Phone the women in your area and find out what their opinions on local hospitals are. (See Useful Addresses, page 157.)
- Hospitals such as King's College in London provide crêches

where children can be looked after whilst you attend the antenatal clinic. Check what provision your hospital provides for the supervision of small children.

Some questions you may want to ask

- Will the hospital allow your partner to be present throughout the birth – and during a caesarean if necessary?
- Is an anaesthetist on call day and night and therefore able to administer an epidural if you decide to have one?
- Can your baby stay with you or go to a nursery at night?
- What are the visiting hours?
- Is there a special baby care unit?
- Can you breastfeed your baby immediately after birth?
- Is it the hospital's policy to remove your baby for 24 hours after birth for observation. This is very common with diabetic mothers' babies and is not always necessary. If the baby is perfectly healthy ask if you can keep him with you.
- What is the usual stay in hospital for a diabetic mother? If the birth goes well there is no reason why you should have to stay in longer than anyone else.
- If you are a vegetarian or have other dietary requirements apart from diabetic ones, check that the hospital can cater for them.
- Many routine practices such as the shaving of pubic hair and the administration of an enema have been rigorously challenged in the last few years and are now not quite as common as they used to be. The removal of pubic hair has been linked to an increase in infection and certainly causes extreme discomfort for the new mother. Ask the staff what their views are on this, and let your own desires be known. I did not experience either thankfully.

If you are part way through your pregnancy and are unhappy about the treatment from your local hospital or the doctors assigned to you, you can change hospitals – you have a right to do this. The happier you are with your pregnancy, the more confident you will feel when you come to deliver the baby. If you are concerned about any aspect of your treatment, talk to your GP about it; if he or she is unsympathetic, then change GPs. Talk to another diabetic woman about the problems you are encountering. Phone someone from the Diabetic Pregnancy Network. Ask to speak to someone in the Care Department at the British Diabetic Association – they will be able to advise you.

The ward timetable

Be prepared. Rest and relaxation isn't something that comes easily in hospital, especially with a routine that goes something like this:

- 6.30 am   The day starts with a cup of tea
- 7.45 am   Blood-glucose test and insulin
- 8 am   Breakfast
- 10–11 am   Blood-glucose test, followed by coffee and biscuits
- 12.00 noon Lunch
- 2–3 pm   Blood-glucose test
- 3 pm   Tea and biscuits
- 5.45 pm   Blood-glucose test and insulin
- 6 pm   Supper
- 9 pm   Blood-glucose test followed by a hot drink

Most hospitals operate a similar day.

Private hospitals

This can mean a hospital which only takes private patients, or an NHS hospital with private rooms which are paid for by its patients. However the cost can be enormous. As well as the obstetrician's fee you must allow for the cost of *all* tests, including scans, drugs and an anaesthetist's services if he is present. Added to this is the possible extra cost of a caesarean and the charge for each night spent in hospital. You should allow at least £2,000. Private medical insurance does not normally cover the cost of a diabetic birth and even if it does, the insurance premiums are very expensive.

If you are able to follow this route the process is as follows.

- Find out which hospitals have the kind of care you are looking for. You can get some information from the *Directory of Private Hospitals and Health Services* published by Medical Market Information Ltd. Your local library should have a copy.
- Talk to your GP about this possibility and ask him to refer

you to a consultant who practises privately.

The problem with private care for the pregnant diabetic apart from the cost is that you need to see two consultants – one who will look after your diabetes and one who will care for your pregnancy. It is important that these two consultants continually liaise with each other. Therefore it would make sense if you could see them both at the same hospital or rooms. If you locate a private diabetic consultant first, ask him to advise you about an obstetrician. This may sound complicated, but it can work.

THE ANTENATAL CLINIC

Many hospitals operate joint antenatal and diabetic clinics. This means less journeying for the patient, with both appointments taking place on the same day. Both clinics will monitor the health of the mother and fetus quite carefully. The following tests are part of that care programme.

Amniocentesis
This is a method of testing for about 40 different possible abnormalities in the baby, including spina bifida and Down's syndrome (mongolism). It is used in association with an ultrasound scan. Amniocentesis is more commonly used in women over 35.

You are first given a pain-killing injection in the lower part of the abdomen. A needle is then inserted into the mother's abdominal wall and into the uterus. A fluid is drawn out through the needle, containing cast-off cells from the fetus, which can then be grown on cell culture plates in the laboratory and analysed.

The **advantages** of an amniocentesis are that:

- It detects abnormalities in the fetus.
- It can reassure older mothers worried about abnormalities.

However, the **disadvantages** are that:

- Between 1 and 2 per cent of mothers miscarry as a result of the test.

- Occasionally the amniocentesis needle causes injury to the baby if the exact position of the fetus has not been properly determined.
- The test cannot be done until you are 16 weeks' pregnant.
- You may be left with a painful bruise.

I did not have an amniocentesis, as this was not thought necessary. Every woman when told she needs to have one should think carefully about this.

Alphafetoprotein (AFP)

This test is done routinely from blood samples taken from the mother's arm. It tests the level of alphafetoprotein (a substance produced by the developing embryo and fetus) which passes into the amniotic fluid and from there into your blood. There is no level which clearly defines an abnormal pregnancy and AFP concentration varies, increasing steadily until it reaches the maximum level at about 30 weeks. It is usually measured between the sixteenth and eighteenth week, the time when the gap between normal and high levels of AFP is greatest.

The **advantages** of the test are that:

- A high level may mean you are later in pregnancy than you thought.
- If AFP is high it may mean you are carrying more than one baby.

There are no disadvantages that I know of. Ask your doctor about the result.

Ultrasound scans

These use high-frequency sound waves which you or your baby cannot hear. They are produced by an object similar to a hairdryer which is run over your abdomen, above the womb. The ultrasound waves bounce off the fetus and show up as a pattern of dots tracing the shape of the baby on a screen – they can even show movement, both of the baby itself and of the fetal heart. The whole thing takes about 10 minutes.

The **advantages** of ultrasound scans are as follows:

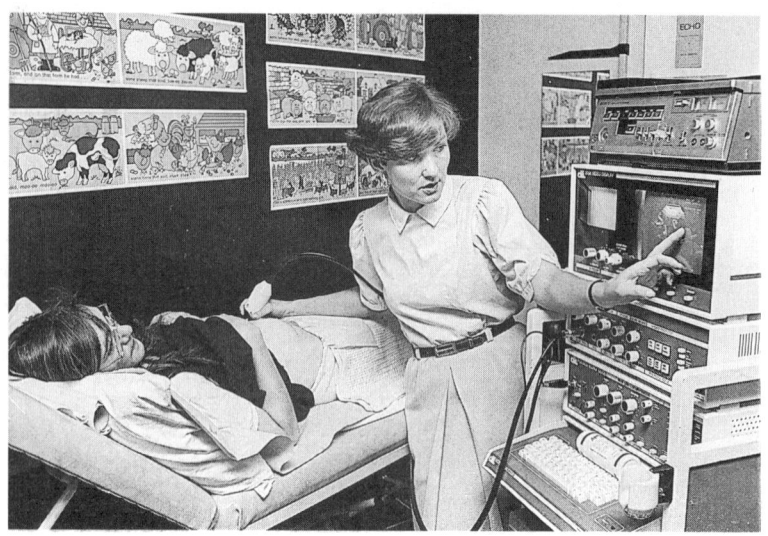

Ultrasound scan being performed.

- Scans detect abnormalities in the fetus. The fetal heartbeat and movement of the baby can be seen.
- They detect the size of the baby by taking very precise measurements, e.g. around the head, the length of arms, etc.
- The baby's development can be assessed.
- Quite often ultrasound scans reassure women who are worried about their pregnancies.
- For the diabetic woman they are particularly advantageous as they can determine the weight of the baby and predict a date when the baby is due.
- They help facilitate bonding with your baby. Once you have seen him kicking and moving around on the screen you may feel very much closer to him than before.

I had four scans throughout my pregnancy; some diabetic women have more, a few less. All the women who wrote to me had experienced them and none showed concern regarding them.

The **disadvantage** of ultrasound scans is that we can be fairly sure that they are safe but not 100 per cent certain. In fact tests done on ultrasound scans suggest there are no hidden dangers, but some women worry none the less.

HPL or human placental lactogen
HPL is a hormone produced by the placenta and found in the mother's blood in increasing amounts as a pregnancy progresses.

It can be tested for by a single blood sample (although a series of tests over two to three weeks is preferred), the result is available in a few hours, and its level can be used to assess the health of the placenta and hence the baby. Low levels after 32 weeks' gestation may indicate fetal distress, small-for-dates babies or a higher chance of a stillbirth.

Oestriol
This is another hormone secreted by the placenta and found circulating in the mother's bloodstream. Its level is estimated by a series of urine samples or blood samples from the mother.

Low levels of the hormone may also indicate fetal distress and an underweight baby, as well as the chance of a stillbirth.

Amniotic fluid analysis
This test is carried out in exactly the same way as an amniocentesis (page 22), although at a later stage in the pregnancy. However, in this test the amniotic fluid itself, rather than the cells suspended in it, is examined.

Diabetic mothers are more at risk of delivering a baby that develops respiratory distress syndrome, particularly if they haven't kept a good control of their blood-glucose levels during pregnancy (see pages 12-13). Amniotic fluid analysis is of particular importance in the assessment of the maturity of the fetal lungs and thus the risks of the baby developing respiratory distress syndrome after birth.

Urine tests for ketones
Ketones are found in the urine when proteins and fats have been broken down in the body. These ketones spill over into the urine from the blood, and they signify that your diabetic control is not good and must be restabilised.

Test strips are used to test urine for ketones. Your doctor will use the test throughout your pregnancy, and he may also ask you to do the test at home.

RENAL THRESHOLD

The renal threshold is the level at which sugars leak over from the bloodstream, via the kidneys, into the urine.

During pregnancy this level may be lower than usual – referred to as a fall in the renal threshold. However, this fall does not mean there is a problem with either the pregnancy or with the baby.

PRE-ECLAMPSIA (TOXAEMIA)

This occasionally occurs in the last half of pregnancy – normally in the seventh to ninth months. It is less common in diabetic women than it used to be, but it is still more likely to be found in diabetic women than amongst the general population.

The symptoms are well recognised; the mother's blood pressure rises, sometimes very rapidly, as the disease progresses, and she will retain water and salt and become oedematous – have swollen legs, ankles, face and hands – and protein will appear in the urine on testing. Despite this, the mother usually feels well and is unaware of the dangers. In the severest cases – true eclampsia – convulsions, coma and maternal and fetal deaths can occur.

The standard view of pre-eclampsia is that it is a disease of unknown origin, the only effective cure being to deliver the baby and the placenta as early as is feasible. Some nutritionists, however, believe that the condition is linked to an inadequate diet – one that is low in protein and essential vitamins and minerals.

Gail Sforza Brewer, one of America's leading childbirth educators, and Dr Tom Brewer, who has done extensive work on the subject of pre-eclampsia and nutrition, have published an informative book which includes details about this disease, entitled *What Every Pregnant Woman Should Know*. It is well worth reading.

Pre-eclampsia is less common if near-normal blood-glucose concentrations are achieved and maintained during the nine months of pregnancy.

WHAT TO EXPECT

The first three months

A missed period is often the first clear sign that conception has occurred and a pregnancy has started. Dates are then calculated by counting from the first day of the last period, up to about 40 weeks. A doctor should be consulted as soon as a pregnancy is suspected. Blood sugar should be tested as often as required and kept within the normal range of 5–8 mmol.

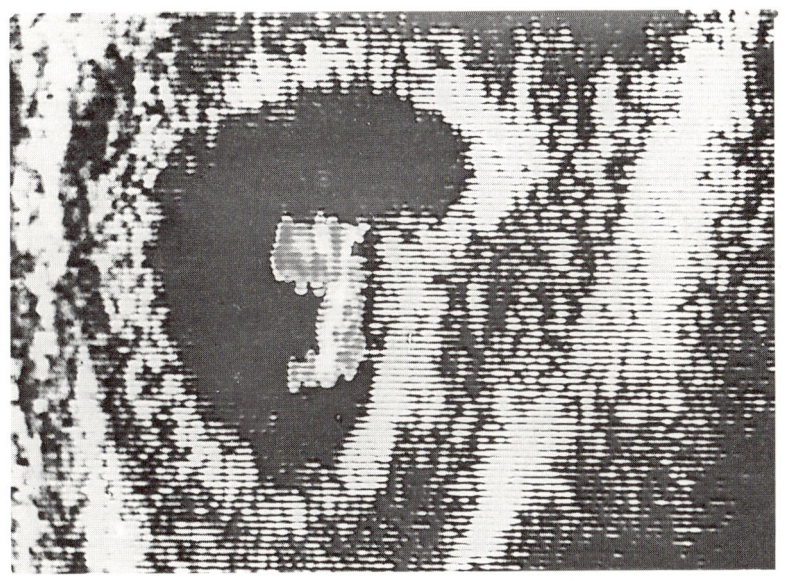

Ultrasound scan of fetus after nine weeks.

Morning sickness may be hard to control as frequent small amounts of carbohydrate, often recommended as a method of combating it, can be difficult to allow for in the course of the usual diabetic diet. The diet itself should include plenty of protein, fresh fruit and vegetables, as well as high-fibre carbohydrate. Unnecessary drugs should be avoided, along with smoking and drinking.

At one month after conception the baby's tiny heart is already beating, and by six weeks the arms and legs have begun to develop. The first sense the baby develops is that of touch, and it is thought that a baby will react to light stroking

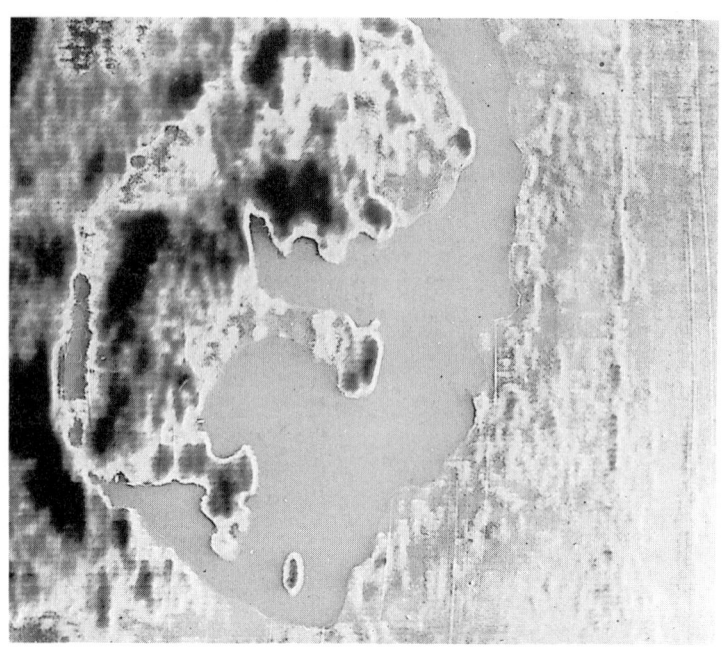

Ultrasound scan of fetus after 12 weeks.

of the womb once it has enlarged enough to be felt above the rim of the pelvis – about 12 weeks after conception. Certainly, many couples instinctively stroke the abdomen, which is thought to be reassuring and pleasurable for the baby.

Creams high in vitamin E can be rubbed onto the abdomen and these may help prevent stretch marks, even though your pregnancy will not be very noticeable at this stage.

The second three months

By this stage the abdominal muscles will have started to relax more, in preparation for the growing baby. Some people find they frequently need to go to the loo as more pressure is exerted on the bladder. The breasts will be growing and may ache occasionally; a good bra will support them and help to maintain their shape. Fluttering may be felt in the lower abdomen – the baby's first movements.

At 12 weeks the baby's sexual organs will be clearly defined

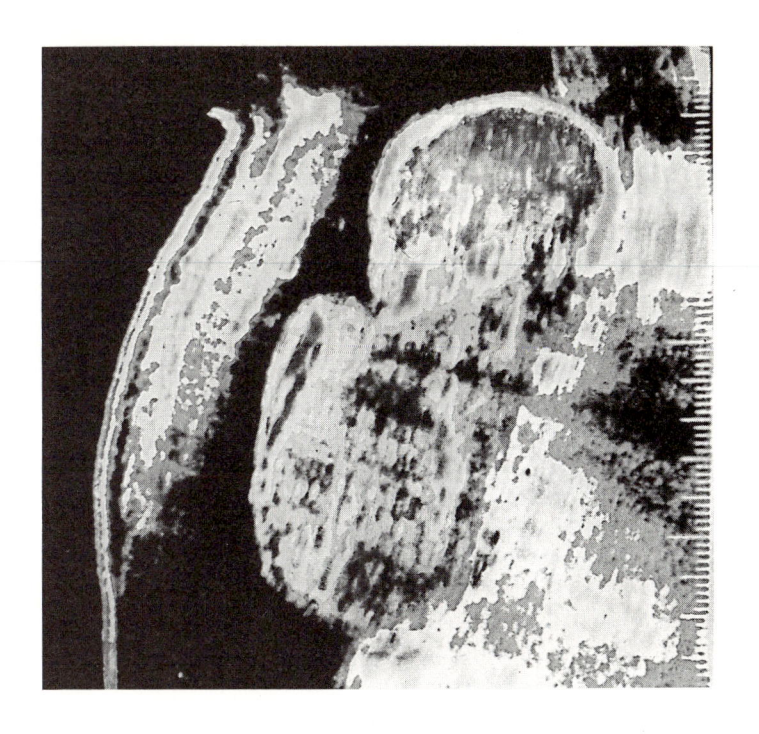

Ultrasound scan of fetus after 21 weeks.

and the fingernails and toenails will be growing. The eyes and nostrils will still be closed, however. The first ultrasound scan will normally take place at around 16–18 weeks.

At five months the baby will be developing very quickly. He will be able to suck, grip and occasionally cough and hiccup, and his hearing mechanism will also be complete.

By the end of six months the baby should be able to hear all the internal sounds made by the mother's body, including the heart beating and the sounds made by the digestive process. The voice of the mother and other members of the family can be heard inside the womb.

The last three months

The pregnancy will be very noticeable by now. Some discomfort may result from the extra weight being carried. Difficulty in sleeping properly is a common problem during this stage of pregnancy.

At 28 weeks the fetal heart can be heard clearly using an ordinary fetal stethoscope. Around the seven-month stage the eyelids will open, enabling the baby to look around and survey his surroundings. The baby will sleep and wake at different times. He is now fully formed but thin and unable to suck properly.

Another ultrasound scan will probably be performed to determine the rate of progress at around 32 weeks' gestation. Visits to the antenatal and diabetic clinic may increase and occur every two weeks from now on. From 36 weeks, visits to the antenatal clinic will be weekly. The baby will continue to put weight on and at around 36 weeks will weigh approximately 5 lb 4 oz (2.4 kg). By this stage he should be in the correct head-down position for birth.

By 40 weeks the baby should have moved down further into the pelvis. This sometimes eases pressure on the abdomen as the head engages (moves down into the pelvis for birth), but unfortunately the pressure on the bladder can often increase and you may well get more tired as a consequence of frequent trips to the loo throughout the night, as well as frequent movement by the baby.

During the last couple of months you may be asked to keep your blood-glucose level lower than normal. This is to prevent the baby becoming too large in the last stages of pregnancy. I aimed to keep my blood-glucose level below 5 mmol and managed it quite easily.

TESTS IN LATE PREGNANCY

Special tests will take place routinely in late pregnancy.

Blood test
This will be performed to check that anaemia has not occurred since the last test. Rhesus antibodies will also be tested for in the case of women who are rhesus negative.

Hormone tests
These tests – HPL and oestriol (see page 25) – will confirm that the placenta is working properly and is continuing to nourish the baby. An induction may follow if the results of this test indicate that the placenta is failing.

POSTNATAL CHECK-UP

Before you leave hospital an appointment will be made for you to return to the clinic for a postnatal check-up. This usually takes place six weeks after the delivery.
At the postnatal check-up:

- The nurse will weigh you.
- A urine sample will be taken to check kidney function.
- Blood pressure will be measured.
- Blood glucose will be tested.

Tell the doctor if you are experiencing any of the following problems:

- Haemorrhoids (piles) – these are quite common following childbirth.
- Stress incontinence – peeing when laughing, sneezing or coughing.
- Depression.
- Pain, following an episiotomy or tear during the delivery.

The doctor will also check:

- That the uterus has involuted, i.e. has returned to its normal non-pregnant size and shape.
- That an episiotomy has healed properly.
- That varicose veins have not appeared.
- That your diabetic control is good.
- That contraceptive measures have been discussed and availability explained should you need them.

MISCARRIAGE

Of all pregnancies, 15 to 20 per cent end in miscarriage, i.e. loss of the fetus before 28 weeks. It is always a deeply upsetting experience for any mother-to-be to lose her baby – even the use of the word 'lose' in such an emotive setting is perhaps a very difficult thing to understand and deal with. Many women suffer intense depression as a result of miscarriage and the thought that this may be nature's way of dealing with a malformed fetus frequently offers little succour. Even very early miscarriages which occur at eight to ten weeks' gestation can be very traumatic for the mother and make early pregnancy in the future an anxious time.

Research has shown that more boys than girls are born each year, but this incidence is reduced somewhat by the fact that more male fetuses are miscarried than female. The reasons for this statistic are unknown.

Miscarriage may be more likely if any of the following circumstances occur.

- Spotting of blood or any bleeding. This is generally treated as a sign that a miscarriage is threatening. The spotting of blood may also be accompanied by pain. If this occurs a doctor should be alerted immediately. Bed rest has always been the recommended action to take, although recent research suggests that this has little effect in preventing a miscarriage.
- Severe cramps or pain. If this incapacitates the woman then it may be indicating the onset of a miscarriage – again the doctor should be called immediately.
- Any sickness, high temperature, severe headache or urinary infection should be dealt with immediately.

Diabetes which is well controlled before conception may not offer any protection from miscarriage during pregnancy, but badly-controlled diabetes will adversely affect the health of the mother and child, perhaps causing the woman to be more susceptible to a miscarriage. The reasons for miscarriage, however, may have nothing to do with being insulin dependent, as this following account demonstrates.

> I had some spotting so I went along to the hospital and they gave me a scan. They found no fetal heartbeat; also the baby had not grown that much since they last looked at eight weeks. This time I was 12 weeks. The doctor told me I would probably miscarry within two days. I did that night. I went straight into hospital.
>
> We were very upset, especially as my levels were always well controlled and my diet included lots of fresh vegetables and high-fibre carbohydrate. I did everything right and it didn't work out. The doctor told me the wrong amount of

chromosomes probably formed at conception, which explains why the baby wasn't growing.

Susan

However, most women who have suffered a miscarriage go on to have a completely normal pregnancy and birth.

When I became pregnant last year for a third time I just decided to be as relaxed as possible, which is very difficult after having lost two babies, and I did think I was going to miscarry for a third time. Instead of lying down in bed for two weeks trying to save my baby, I went about my everyday business and was thrilled to give birth to a beautiful baby boy.

Lesley

The upsetting experience of miscarriage can have long-lasting effects and many women take a great deal of time to recover from one. Talk to other women and gain support from them. You may be surprised by the number who have shared the same feelings.

There are no reasons to suggest that a miscarriage can happen as a result of sexual intercourse during pregnancy or a minor accident such as a fall. Some women have been prescribed folic acid daily and often the addition of vitamin E has led to successful births. A diet rich in yeast, wheatgerm and green leafy vegetables will provide adequate amounts of folic acid.

Premature labour

If you start to go into labour between about 26–8 weeks and 36 weeks this is known as premature or early labour. It should be distinguished from miscarriage: miscarriage invariably means that the baby does not survive; in premature labour there is an increasing chance of the baby surviving, especially later in the pregnancy.

It is imperative that you should contact the hospital or your midwife if the following occur:

- The waters break. Leakage of amniotic fluid may cause labour to start prematurely. Any continued leakage which follows a sudden flow of fluid should be reported to the

hospital. After 36 weeks the breaking of waters is less important as the baby has a greater chance of survival.
- Any bleeding of fresh or old blood, however small.
- The onset of any continued contractions – often felt as severe cramps or pains.
- Absence of fetal movements. If the baby has not moved for longer than 24 hours then a doctor should be contacted. Some women keep a detailed kick-chart in the later weeks of pregnancy. The sleeping and waking patterns can then be gauged quite easily and can be used to allay fears.

4

MAINTAINING BALANCE

HOME BLOOD-GLUCOSE MEASUREMENTS

A comprehensive record of home blood-glucose tests kept throughout pregnancy will be the most valuable aid for both the doctor and the patient. It will provide a clear picture of the body's need for insulin and will enable good diabetic control for the full nine-month period. The purpose of these home blood-glucose measurements is:

- To detect hyperglycaemia and hypoglycaemia.
- To measure changes of blood glucose during a 24-hour period. The tests will give a blood-glucose profile, showing where the peaks and troughs occur. The profile will also demonstrate the duration, or action, of different insulins on individual patients. This varies a great deal from person to person.
- To assess blood-glucose control in times of special need so that insulin dosages can be readjusted accordingly.

Obtaining a blood-glucose profile

To obtain a full blood-glucose profile blood samples should be taken at the following times:

- Before the morning injection
- 1½–2 hours after breakfast
- Before lunch
- 1½–2 hours after lunch
- Before the evening injection
- 1½–2 hours after the evening meal

- Before bedtime
- At some point during the night

Try, if possible, to do two home profiles before visits to the diabetic clinic or doctor in charge of your diabetes – it will give him or her a clearer picture of what is happening.

If you feel your control has not been as good as it might have been it may be tempting occasionally to alter the results in order to please your doctor. I know in a lot of clinics patients are made to feel like naughty children if results are less than satisfactory. However, it is best not to walk along this particular road – it is heavily mined. The co-operation between patient and doctor is vital at all times and honesty can only further a good working relationship. Blood sugar will rise at certain points during pregnancy due to the extra demands made on your body by the baby. The doctor needs to know this, so that insulin dosage can be altered.

If you are unable to do full profiles at home then test before breakfast, before lunch, before dinner and at bedtime, and

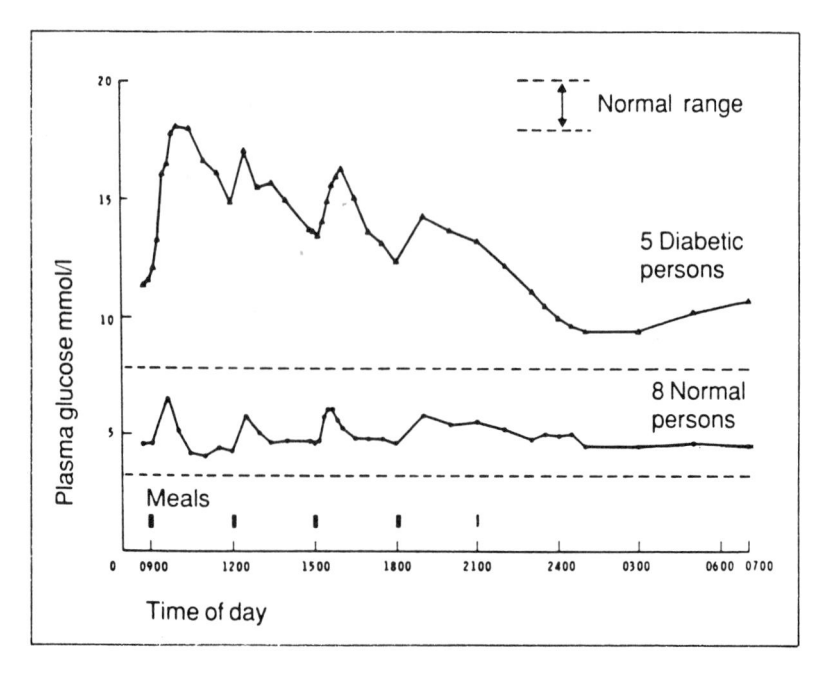

Blood-glucose profile showing fluctuations throughout the day.

make a note of the results. The more often you do test for blood glucose, the more detailed the profile will be.

Glycosylated haemoglobin (HbA₁)
This test (see page 8) will be done a few times at the clinic. It will measure average control over the last six-week period.

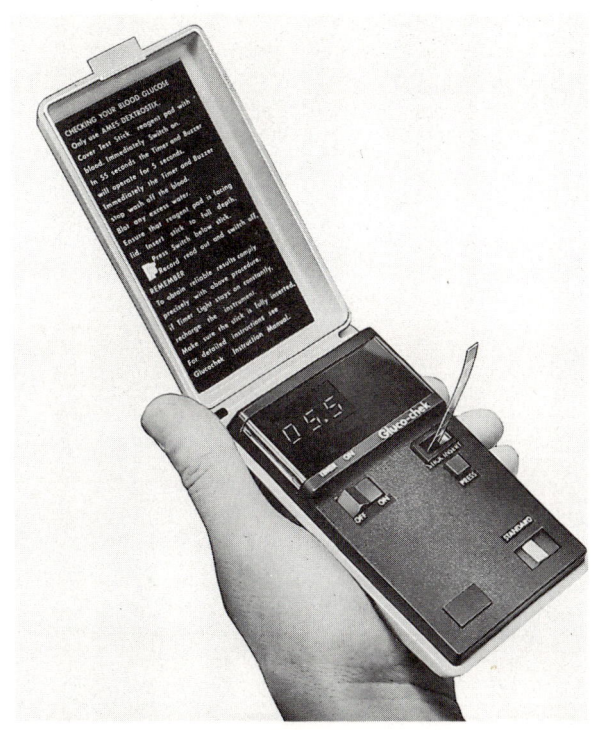

Blood-glucose monitoring meter.

Blood-glucose monitoring meters
These meters are designed to measure the amount of glucose in the blood and give an exact reading. The finger is pricked and blood put onto a test strip. The strip is inserted into a little computer and the timer activated. The reading will then appear on a large legible panel.

The **advantages** of meters are that:

- The readings given are more accurate than the traditional visual test strip.

- The result is easier to read.
- They are fairly portable – about the size of a paperback book.
- Some people enjoy using them so much they test their blood sugar far more than they would normally.

However there are **disadvantages**:

- They can be very expensive – anything upwards of £50. Some hospitals will, however, lend a computer to a woman who is pregnant.
- The meters have to be well maintained in order to operate properly.

All meters are accurate provided the manufacturers' instructions are adhered to exactly.

Telemetry

Some hospitals are using computers in a slightly different way in order to keep a check on blood-sugar levels. Patients take their blood-glucose readings at home four to six times a day and these are recorded automatically on their home meters. Once a week these home meter-readings are transferred via their phone lines into the hospital computer. The hospital computer printouts containing all the information are then shown to the doctors, who will phone a patient back immediately if they feel that it is necessary to alter the insulin dosage.

The **advantages** of this system are that:

- Where transport is a problem this is a time-saving way of getting the doctor to oversee your control of your blood-glucose levels.
- It is a particularly advantageous system for pregnant women who are testing their blood sugars frequently.

Ask your doctor if this system is available in your area – it most often works where a large hospital serves many towns and small outlying villages.

INSULIN

During pregnancy, diabetes will be balanced using insulin. Insulin is either extracted from pigs and cows for use with humans, or human insulin is engineered genetically, using the DNA technique.

There are two distinct types of insulin that the body requires, clear insulin and cloudy insulin. Ask your doctor to explain the exact action of the insulin you are using, as so many different ones are now used.

Clear insulin
This insulin, also known as short-acting insulin, acts quickly when injected and has a limited duration of activity – it lasts up until about 8 hours. It is absorbed quickly and if it is injected in the morning it will reach a peak an hour or two after breakfast.

Cloudy insulin
This insulin acts more slowly. It will usually last for between 12 to 14 hours. It keeps the blood-glucose level stable between meals and is often referred to as long-acting insulin.

Amount of insulin
Almost all women who have diabetes and are pregnant will be asked to take two injections per day. These injections will consist of a set amount of clear insulin and, generally, a larger amount of cloudy insulin. The dose will be supervised by a doctor, but many people alter their own dosage according to home blood-glucose readings.

During the latter half of pregnancy, the body's need for insulin increases, due to the hormonal changes that are occurring. This does not indicate that the diabetes is worsening in any way. Because of this, some women are advised to have three or more injections a day in order to achieve the desired control.

Insulin pens
Insulin pens received a lot of praise from the women who wrote to me, who used them very happily throughout pregnancy.

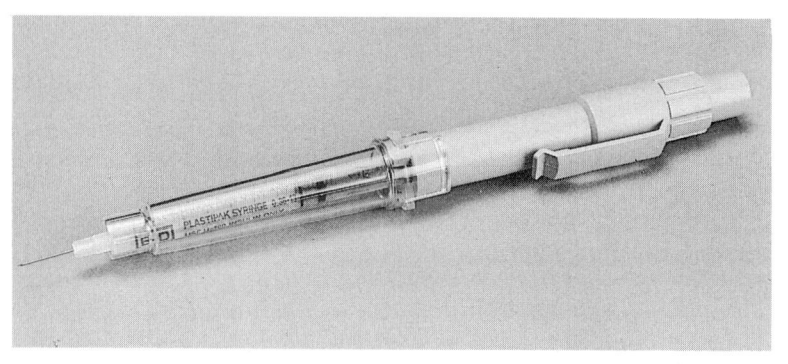

Insulin pen.

However, these pens should only be used under the advice of a doctor.

With an insulin pen, clear short-acting insulin is injected during the day, using the pen half an hour before meals. One injection of cloudy longer-acting insulin is then given before bed, using a traditional syringe.

The **advantages** of insulin pens are that:

- Mealtimes can occur at whatever time you want. For example, breakfast can be at 11 am, lunch can be missed out and you can have dinner when you are hungry. The system allows for a far greater flexibility of lifestyle than using a syringe all the time.
- The size of meals can vary.
- Insulin is already drawn up and available in the pen, so saving time.
- The pens actually resemble writing pens and can be used discreetly, e.g. on aeroplanes and at restaurant tables.

However there are **disadvantages** to insulin pens:

- The pens can cost over £30 to purchase, and are not available on the NHS, even though the insulin that is used in the pens is available on prescription just the same as any other insulin.
- It is best to have two pens available, in case one is mislaid or lost – a traditional syringe cannot be used with the insulin designed for specific use with the pen.

Recent research has shown that diabetic control when using a pen is no better or worse than control using the usual syringe system, although people using the pens have noticed that a much more flexible and normal eating routine can be introduced. However, all the women who praised the insulin pens in letters to me did test their blood glucose regularly and were able to alter dosages quite easily. It can take a few weeks to become confident enough in your own control to use a pen effectively.

Insulin infusion pumps

These pumps are either worn on a belt around the waist or on a shoulder holster. They work by providing a small continuous flow of insulin throughout the day. A spurt of insulin just before a meal can be triggered by the wearer. A needle is permanently situated in the skin under the abdomen, and this receives the insulin from the pump.

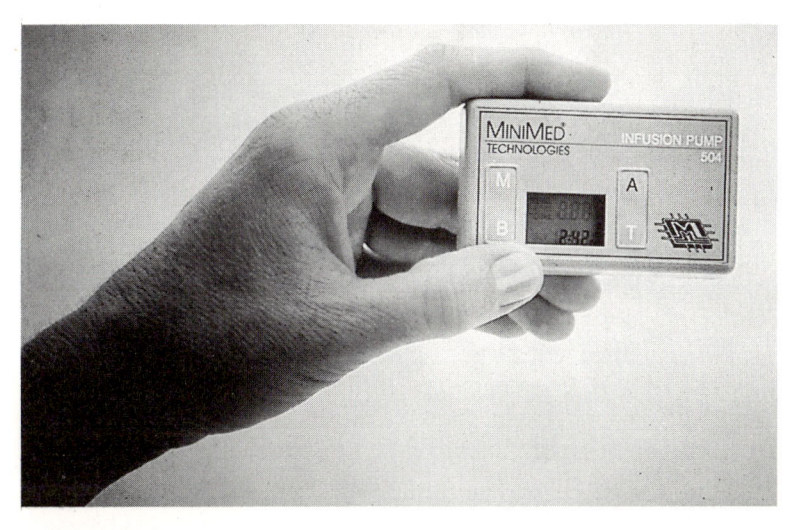

Insulin infusion pump.

Pumps are only used when the diabetes is difficult to control by any other method. They have now achieved a slightly unfashionable status and are not used as much. Their **advantages** are that:

- Some people treat them with the same joy and curiosity as

they would a computer toy, and enjoy using them enormously.
- Meals can be eaten at the desired times, and the amounts of food eaten can be varied.
- Some people achieve good control using them.

The **disadvantages** of insulin pumps are that:

- They are cumbersome and noticeable.
- Pump failures and malfunctions are frequent, in some cases causing serious consequences.
- Frequent monitoring and maintenance of the pump is required.
- There are a variety of models, and some can be very expensive to purchase.
- The pump must be removed for bathing, sport and sexual intercourse. Afterwards the needle must then be reinserted.
- Pumps are not available on the NHS.

HYPOGLYCAEMIA – VERY LOW BLOOD SUGAR

Unless we understand how our bodies react in everyday circumstances, unforeseen problems can occur. Knowing how you feel at all times is the most important aspect of being able to recognise the early signs of having a hypo. If you don't smoke or drink or take any other substances which alter the way you feel, then detecting the first symptoms of a hypo should be easy.

Throughout each and every day, if any feelings of queasiness occur, then ask yourself if this is the first stage of a hypo, or merely something else. You will experience some of the following if your blood sugar is low:

- Unusual dizziness
- Hunger
- Nausea
- Paleness of skin
- Headache

These are clear signs of an insulin reaction – a hypo – and are fairly easy to detect. Glucose or something sweet should be taken immediately. If these symptoms aren't treated quickly, then the following may occur:

- Trembling
- Confusion
- Odd behaviour
- Loss of consciousness

Having a hypo

The initial symptoms may vary considerably from person to person. Some people are aware of a low blood sugar immediately, whilst others find it difficult to make an assessment.

The experience of having a serious hypo is an extremely unnerving one, although it can have a very seductive effect on the mental processes. I remember frequently waking in the past with a hypo and thinking about incredibly interesting subjects in an extraordinary way. The brain, when it is so animated, provides a great deal of entertainment, to the extent that I have often been loathe to end the hypo. Of course it is always vital to do so, and earlier rather than later, but it can be difficult trying to make a non-hypoglycaemic decision.

Often sufferers of a severe hypo refuse glucose and sugar and become very difficult to manage. The part of the brain that has been trained to say no to sweet items of food is now being expected to shut down. Frequently I can remember refusing to drink something sweet, thinking the liquid would send my blood sugar soaring, and I would pretend to behave like a fully-controlled human in order to get the person trying to administer the glucose to take it away. My husband and I made an agreement, after a few of these exasperating occasions, that I would always take the glucose at night if he thought my blood glucose was down. He has so far never been wrong, and since the agreement hypos at night, although infrequent, are handled with greater ease. Somehow the agreement has erased my stubbornness, causing my subconscious to honour it.

When I do experience hypos during the day I am easily able to detect them. I always ask myself a checklist of questions when I feel my blood glucose may be low and test it as soon as possible. Years ago I went through a period of total nontesting and it led to all sorts of dramas, including being found one morning trying to peer behind the wallpaper and carefully undoing it at the seams in order to facilitate this delicate operation.

Once when my blood glucose was extremely low I left my husband in a restaurant in Greece and went next door into a small supermarket to get some shopping. I was in the shop for about an hour. I remember picking up all the packets of biscuits and squeezing them so that the biscuits inside disintegrated. Laughing like a hyena, I was then happily placing the ruined contents back on the shelves. I must have done this to about 20 packets. One side of my brain obviously realised at some juncture that I needed carbohydrate, but the other side was used to refusing such items of food, with the consequence that I was handling the desired glucose but not actually consuming it.

Thankfully, my husband decided to look for me and shouted through the glass window to hurry up. He then sat outside on a motorbike that we had hired that day. Like an escapee from a mental hospital, I grabbed armfuls of chocolate and ran out of the shop, past the till and various customers as well as the Greek owners, and jumped onto the bike. Dave drove up the road, whilst inquiring whether I had paid for this armful of food I was littering the road with. I couldn't answer this as I was unable to stop giggling for long enough. Eventually he stopped, realised what was happening and shoved some food in my mouth.

Later on when I realised I could have been slung into jail for shoplifting, I was horrified. I wasn't carrying any identification or personal details whatsoever. After a day on the beach, where I was feeling quite lightheaded, I had totally mistaken the symptoms of hypoglycaemia and assumed them to be the effects of too much sun and retsina.

That particular incident is possibly the worst of its kind and serves as a clear reminder of how important it is to take care of your own diabetes so that the responsibilities of it aren't shouldered by other people.

SOLUTIONS TO HYPOGLYCEMIA

Glucose tablets

If these are easily available then time will not have to be spent searching. Some women have found during pregnancy that the early warning signs of hypoglycaemia rapidly move onto loss of consciousness without very much time in between. It is better to take glucose unnecessarily at these times than to risk hypoglycemia.

- Put glucose tablets under your pillow at night.
- Put a packet in your handbag.
- Leave some in the glove compartment of your car.
- Put them in an accessible place at work.
- *Never go anywhere without some.*

Many women carry mini Mars bars or other attractive sugary items in case of an emergency. In my own experience, it is more common that I will imagine a hypo if I am in the vicinity of such foods. Glucose tablets are not likely to be eaten at the wrong time, whereas sweets and other sugary things are, often to excess.

Check your blood sugar soon after a hypo to make sure that glucose levels have been restored – four or five glucose tablets should be enough. Then take some longer-lasting carbohydrate to see you through to the next meal or injection – toast or a sandwich will usually suffice.

Glucagon

Some women experience unexpected severe attacks of hypoglycaemia during pregnancy, which can cause unconsciousness. In such circumstances glucagon can be administered, for example by a partner or a friend.

Glucagon consists of a hormone which can be injected. It restores your blood sugar to normal very quickly, allowing you to regain consciousness. Then, when you have recovered, you should take some carbohydrate to prevent another reaction occurring.

How to administer glucagon.

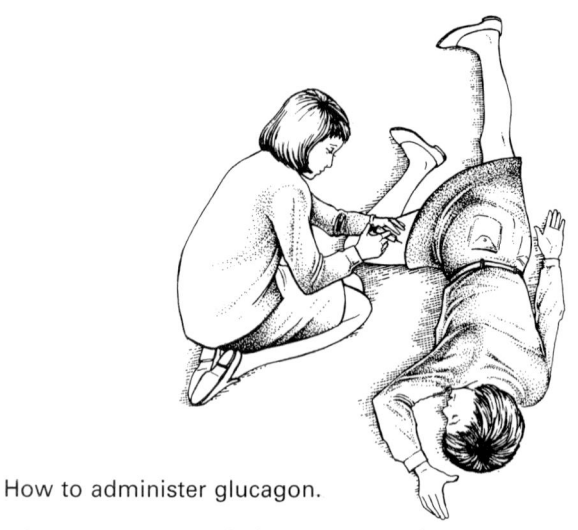

The **advantages** of glucagon are that:

- You and your partner will feel more secure knowing you have this available in emergencies.
- It can be administered quickly.
- It is perfectly safe to use.
- It can be stored in the fridge.

However there are **disadvantages**:

- The procedure to follow in order to give a glucagon injection is slightly complicated, so the user needs to be fully aware of the steps to take. Your doctor will show you.
- Some people may rely on it too heavily, thereby not taking sufficient care with their blood glucose.
- If your partner is squeamish about injections then he probably will not be able to give you glucagon.

Hypostop

This is a fast-acting dextrose in gel form. It consists of a thick clear jelly which can be easily administered and absorbed. If you do become unconscious because of a hypo, some Hypostop can simply be squeezed into your mouth and rubbed around inside – you will usually absorb enough to bring you round. Hypostop costs around £1.50 per plastic bottle, and can easily be carried around with you.

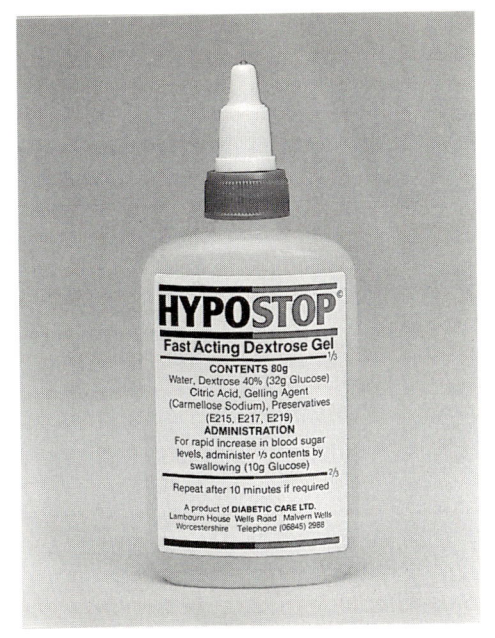

Hypostop.

HYPERGLYCAEMIA

In this condition you have very high blood-sugar levels. It may occur when:

- You contract an infection.
- You overeat.
- You are inactive for long periods of time.
- You forget to take your injection and eat normally.

All diabetic women will have to increase their insulin dosage at certain stages during pregnancy. However, if a sudden and inexplicable rise in your blood sugar takes place then your doctor should be contracted.

If your blood-glucose levels do become raised you will experience some of the following symptoms:

- Frequent trips to the loo
- Extreme thirst
- Tiredness and drowsiness

- Vomiting and nausea
- Headache

Going to the loo frequently is a condition of pregnancy in the later weeks, so cannot be taken as an indication of high blood sugar on its own. You must therefore test your blood glucose as soon as you suspect that it may be rising. Hyperglycaemia takes longer to develop than low blood sugar but it also takes longer to rectify, so it is important that it is remedied before it is allowed to escalate.

A small dose of fast-acting insulin will usually reduce the level of sugar in your blood fairly quickly. However, if control is good throughout pregnancy, then it will be easier to keep your blood glucose at a steady rate.

YOUR FAMILY AND FRIENDS

Educate your family, friends and colleagues – make sure that those people who are in regular contact with you know that you have diabetes.

- Show them where your glucose tablets are kept.
- Tell them what to look for, so they can identify a hypoglycaemic reaction. If you don't tell them these things who will? It will be a nuisance answering all those extra questions but they may mean help for other people with diabetes in the future.
- Ask your partner to test your blood sugar so that he is as familiar with the process as you are.
- Wear an identification necklace or bracelet such as Medic-Alert at all times.

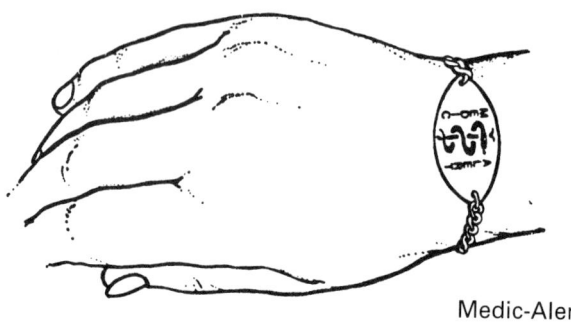

Medic-Alert bracelet.

INFECTIONS

Pregnant women are generally more prone to infections such as thrush, cystitis, etc. In part this is because their immune system (which fights infection) is marginally depressed in order to prevent rejection of the fetus. However, infections of any kind in a diabetic can upset the blood-glucose control, so if you do get an infection you should seek immediate help from your doctor.

One very common ailment amongst diabetic women is thrush. It is caused by a fungal infection of the skin around the vulva, vagina and sometimes the anus, and may recur frequently if your blood glucose is high – the sugary environment is ideal for the growth of this fungus.

The symptoms of thrush are itching and irritation between the legs, often causing an itchy red area to appear, and there is frequently a creamy vaginal discharge. Creams and pessaries are often prescribed; they will cure the infection if used as instructed, but will not prevent thrush from recurring. Some women find an application of live yoghurt onto the irritated skin is very helpful when the symptoms first appear; however this is less helpful if the symptoms have been ignored for a few days. Years ago gentian violet was often applied to the irritated skin, with very good results, but it was an extremely messy procedure and was discontinued for that reason.

To avoid thrush:

- Keep blood-glucose levels normal.
- Avoid wearing tight-fitting clothes such as jeans if you are susceptible to this ailment. (During pregnancy you probably won't want to wear such clothes anyway.)
- Wear cotton underwear.

Other infections such as colds and flu will also alter your blood-glucose levels, and your insulin dosage may have to be increased so that your blood sugar does not rise too high.

WHEN TO CONTACT THE DOCTOR

Always contact your doctor if any of the following occur:

- Sugars rise unusually high or regularly drop extremely low. Insulin dosage may need greater adjustments than you are already making.
- Ketones are detected in the urine. This could mean the diabetes is getting out of control.
- Any illness.
- Symptoms of a bladder infection, such as pain and a burning sensation when going to the loo.
- A noticeable decrease in the baby's movements and kicks.

5

GESTATIONAL DIABETES

Gestational diabetes refers specifically to women who develop diabetes during pregnancy; it affects up to 2.5 per cent of pregnant women.

All mothers-to-be undergo simple routine blood tests for diabetes during pregnancy. If gestational diabetes is diagnosed, it will be treated in exactly the same way as an insulin-dependent diabetic who is also pregnant. The diabetes will be stabilised using insulin injections and the diet will be adjusted as a result of these.

The possibility of gestational diabetes may be suspected if:

- There is a history of diabetes in the family.
- The patient has previously given birth to a large baby, i.e. over 9 lb, (4 kg).
- The woman has suffered a stillbirth in the past.
- There is a history of sugar in the urine or in previous blood tests.
- The mother is overweight.

Gestational diabetes is mainly confirmed in the last three months of pregnancy. The symptoms are:

- Extreme thirst
- Lethargy
- Constant need to urinate
- Loss of weight

These are the same symptoms suffered by any newly-diagnosed diabetic.

Immediately after birth the blood glucose of the mother will be tested. About 98 per cent of mothers will return to normal and no longer require the use of insulin. However approximately 30 per cent will develop diabetes within the next five years, and 60 per cent will probably develop diabetes within the next 10 years.

The only action a woman can take in order to prevent this eventual onslaught of the disease is to keep the body weight down. This does not automatically protect someone from developing the disease, but bearing in mind the fact that diabetes is generally more common in people who are overweight, it may certainly help.

Although the gestational diabetes may disappear once the baby is born, it can recur with subsequent pregnancies. Your doctor should be alerted once a further pregnancy is suspected.

It is important once gestational diabetes has been diagnosed to keep the blood-glucose levels within the 5–8 mmol spectrum. Good control is just as important for the gestational diabetic as it is for the traditional diabetic woman. The aims, of course, are always the same – the birth of a healthy baby of normal weight.

WOMEN'S EXPERIENCES

Here are some first-hand accounts of women who have experienced gestational diabetes, which may help you if you are newly diagnosed.

> I became diabetic in January 1982 when I was about five months' pregnant. I was put on insulin. I started to attend the diabetic clinic on Tuesday morning and on a Wednesday morning I was admitted to the maternity ward for 24 hours for four-hourly blood tests. This became my routine for a couple of months. My first child had just started school.
>
> I expected to have an extremely big baby, around the 12 lb mark (5.5 kg). I also expected to be admitted to hospital for the last four weeks of my confinement and I expected to have an induced labour by caesarean section. I was extremely worried. You tend to bottle things up at times like that, but in my head I kept on wondering whether

my doctors knew what they were doing. I eventually asked my doctor what he intended doing about my pregnancy, and at what stage they would induce me. He told me I was quite healthy and my blood control was good, so he could see no reason why I wouldn't have a normal pregnancy going to full term.

Eventually I went into labour and we called the ambulance at about 5 am on a Wednesday morning. The pains stopped and didn't really start again until visiting time in the evening. I was taken to the delivery suite at about 9 pm. In fact I walked to it. I gave birth at two minutes past 10. There was a doctor in attendance, but all he had to do was watch from a corner of the room. I don't even think he spoke a word. I had no pain-killers, no drugs of any description. The whole episode was so much easier than with my first child, and with her I wasn't diabetic.

By 10.20 I was eating two slices of toast and drinking tea. My little boy weighed 8 lb (3.6 kg) and was perfectly healthy.

Once at home I started to get hypos more and more frequently, so on my visit to the clinic I talked to the doctor and we decided between us that I should come off insulin but keep a check on urine tests. For 10 weeks I was okay but then I found sugar again in my urine. I went back to the hospital and have been on injections ever since.

I live the normal ordinary humdrum life of a housewife. I'm no different to the woman next door. I have two lovely children who are such a handful. My youngest with whom I became diabetic is at playschool at the moment. He starts school in August and is so full of energy, life and mischief, it is unbelievable. A perfect birth and a perfect handful of a four-year-old.

Linda

I had a baby boy 7 lb 9 oz (3.4 kg) on the 30 January this year, but I was only diagnosed diabetic at 12 weeks' pregnant. I was lucky in that my obstetrician had a particular interest in diabetes and I also had an excellent diabetic doctor and liaison nurse. All three worked together throughout my pregnancy.

To begin with I was diet controlled, but my sugar levels did not respond and at five months I became insulin dependent. Fortunately I found it no problem to inject and was able to understand insulin and the actions of the different types. I started on a low dose of human Ultratard and ended up with twice-daily injections of Actrapid and Insultard mixed – taking over 50 units a day at one time. It seemed a lot to me. The size of the baby did not come under 'control' until I started the Actrapid, then all progressed normally until I was 36 weeks. The last two weeks of my pregnancy were hell because although they allowed me to up my insulin, as my readings allowed, they were not keen on the reverse. They were trying for extremely tight control and I hypoed most nights at around 2.00 am when the baby seemed most active.

They and I decided enough was enough and I was induced at 38 weeks – even though the consultant had been very keen for me to go full term! I had the double drip (insulin and glucose). My labour was 4½ hours long and nearly resulted in an emergency caesar as the baby's heartbeat dropped. As it was they gave me an episiotomy to try forceps, but it was not needed as we beat them to it!

During my pregnancy I had a scan every two weeks and hospital visits every two weeks. Luckily I saw the same people and we all became quite friendly. I was lucky to have been well briefed about hypos before.

I had to spend three days in hospital at five months due to an infection caused by the diabetes, and 24 hours for a blood-sugar test.

My diabetes went with the birth and, as it is expected back with another pregnancy, I'm sure the experience I've had will stand me in good stead, particularly if I have the same medical team. I feel I have been very lucky, especially when I look at my lovely happy little boy.

Judith

Although I have three children, only one of my pregnancies was a diabetic one, as I only developed the condition four years ago. At about 22 weeks sugar was discovered in my urine. I hadn't noticed any symptoms of diabetes before (I'm a doctor), so I thought that it was probably a mistake due to my dirty jam jar for containing urine. However, when I repeated the tests at home they were positive as well. My next excuse was that my renal threshold was probably altered because of the pregnancy. My husband (also a doctor) tested my blood sugar, expecting it to be normal but it was about 13 mmol.

The next step was to take a blood-sugar profile over a 24-hour period. I took the result of that to my diabetologist-to-be. I was already on a restricted carbohydrate diet as I suffer from a number of food allergies including, strangely enough, sucrose.

The only time I have problems keeping food down is when I'm pregnant, because of the almost constant nausea I suffer from. So, as we couldn't expect any improvement in my blood sugar from further alteration in diet, I went straight onto insulin. Initially I had two doses of Monotard a day – about eight units. The dose increased as pregnancy progressed and soon Actrapid insulin was given with each injection. I tried to keep my blood-glucose levels below 7 mmol, and found control was easy to maintain. Interestingly enough, hypoglycaemia was not a problem in spite of the nausea.

At 38 weeks I went into hospital for induction. I was not in hospital at all before that. As I was to be induced in the afternoon I had my normal breakfast and soluble insulin. During the morning I was put onto an insulin pump with a simultaneous dextrose infusion. My blood sugar was carefully monitored throughout the day.

The actual labour progressed normally. I had a normal delivery after four hours and a healthy 8½ lb (3.9 kg) girl who was not at all affected by my diabetes.

Linda

I am 33 years old and developed diabetes during my second pregnancy, two years ago. I was 25 weeks' pregnant at the time. I was given a finger-pricking maching, a supply of BM sticks, told how to balance myself and sent home. At first I was at the hospital every three days, then every week, then every two weeks alternating with the antenatal clinic. Throughout the remainder of my pregnancy the diabetic clinic was calm, reasonable and encouraging.

I was due to be induced at 37½ weeks because the baby was large but managed to go into labour myself at 37 weeks and had a normal delivery. My son was 9 lb 6 oz (4.2 kg) – a heavy baby.

After the birth my sugar returned to near normal and I was non-diabetic for 10 weeks, then I started to get thirsty and quite ill and was started back on injections again. This time it took a long time to balance me.

The relief at having a normal, healthy baby was unspeakable. I felt fitter, leaner and found the diabetes less of an inconvenience than I thought.

Alex

ASIAN WOMEN

Asian women living in the West have been found to have a greater incidence of gestational diabetes than any other group. This may be due to the differences in diet or body weight.

Lowering the level of fat consumed is thought to be one way of improving your food intake and limiting calories. Fruit and vegetables, which are often low in our Western diet, and milk and yoghurt, which may provide the major source of the essential vitamin B_{12}, both feature in the balanced vegetarianism practised by Asian cultures. This generally provides an extremely healthy diet, often superior to our own. The cause of gestational diabetes amongst Asian women has not yet been clearly identified.

6

KEEPING HEALTHY

LOOK AFTER YOURSELF

Optimum health during pregnancy cannot be achieved if you smoke or drink. It isn't fair on the developing baby to have to suffer your cigarettes and alcohol.

Cut down on caffeine

Tea and coffee are a normal part of most people's lives, but they do contain caffeine, over-consumption of which can lead to hyperactivity and even birth defects in babies. It has also been suggested that caffeine prevents the proper absorption of the B-complex vitamins. Coca-Cola (including the low-calorie variety), many soft drinks, chocolate and cocoa also contain caffeine, and can bump up a normal caffeine intake.

Caffeine-free coffees and juices are readily available and should be substituted before conception and during pregnancy if possible.

Try to avoid unnecessary drugs

Many abortions are carried out each year because of malformed fetuses due to drugs prescribed by doctors who did not realise their patients were pregnant. If there is the remotest chance that conception may have occurred, tell your doctor. Try not to take drugs for minor complaints such as headache or cold. For example, aspirin has been linked with abnormalities and low birth-weight in babies, while the effects of some other drugs on the fetus are still unknown. Insulin used to control diabetes will not harm the baby; neither will thyroxine and many other necessary drugs. Talk to your doctor if you have any worries.

What else can I do?

- Make sure your family, friends and workmates know what to do if you have a hypo.
- Inform the Driver and Vehicle Licensing Centre at Swansea and your car insurance company that you have diabetes.
- Carry identification, such as a Medic-Alert disc or a card stating that you have diabetes, with you at all times.
- Listen to your body. Rest when you are tired.
- Test your blood glucose if you are feeling unwell.
- Inform your doctor if anything is worrying you. Put yourself first and be aware of your own needs.

DIABETES AND YOUR BODY

In order to achieve and maintain good health we need to be aware of certain conditions which the diabetic of some years' standing is more likely to suffer from.

Damage to the eyes

Minor problems with the eyes are found in 70 per cent of people who have suffered diabetes for longer than 25 years. And more serious problems may occur, such as cataracts, glaucoma, and retinopathy, when the blood vessels at the back of the retina begin to leak blood into the eye. All these conditions can be brought on more swiftly and exacerbated by badly-controlled diabetes.

However, all these problems associated with the eyes of a diabetic can now be treated by eye specialists, often with the use of modern techniques such as lasers. It is therefore very important that your eyes are checked annually by the doctor looking after your diabetes.

Damage to the kidneys

Approximately 25 to 40 per cent of long-standing diabetics (over 25 years) have some problems with kidney function. High blood-glucose readings over a long period increase the chance of kidney disease developing. Sometimes the damage caused to the kidneys may be irreversible and the patient will have to use a kidney dialysis machine in order to live.

A consistently good blood-glucose balance throughout life is the only way to avoid this distressing condition.

Hardening of the arteries

If the arteries become hardened and furred-up, the flow of blood is restricted through them and this blockage can lead eventually to a heart attack or stroke. The incidence of this condition is increasing in the Western world, and is more common amongst diabetics than the population at large. Generally, women are three times less likely to suffer from heart disease than men, but the diabetic woman, unfortunately, does not have this advantage – she is equally at risk from the disease as are any of the male members of society.

The demands of motherhood are such that diabetic control and good eating habits can easily fall into last place in the order of things requiring attention. However, with a little effort a diabetic woman can do something to prevent hardened arteries and heart disease occurring.

- Don't smoke. Not only does smoking interfere with insulin absorption; it also helps to fur up arteries more rapidly.
- Reduce the consumption of cholesterol which is found in high-fat dairy produce and meat. Cholesterol helps to fur up arteries.
- Try to substitute vegetable fats for animal fats. Don't cook, bake or spread bread with lard, butter or high-fat margarine.
- Eat more food that is high in fibre, such as oatmeal, pasta and all kinds of beans. They will actually help to lower the blood-cholesterol levels.
- Exercise – for example, walking three times a week at a fast pace for 20 minutes each time is sufficient.
- Keep your blood glucose within the normal range.

Damage to feet

Nerve damage in the legs and feet is commonly found in diabetics who have had the disease for 25 years or more. This means that damage to the feet may go undetected because of the lack of sensation of pain. Furthermore, poor circulation and slow healing may aggravate such problems. Accidental injuries or minor infections must be treated promptly to prevent the threat of gangrene. Check your feet regularly.

- Keep your feet clean at all times.
- Wear good-fitting comfortable shoes that do not rub or chafe.
- Check footwear for bits of gravel and other objects before you put them on.
- Don't go barefoot.
- Consult a doctor if you notice any corns, ingrowing toenails or cuts which haven't healed properly, as well as any loss of feeling.
- Don't smoke, as cigarettes impair circulation.
- Test bath water carefully, as the ability to detect very hot or very cold water may be dulled.
- Don't use hot-water bottles or electric blankets – these can burn your feet and legs without you noticing.
- Use a moisturising cream on the feet if you suffer from dry skin, or put a few drops of baby oil in the bath water.
- Good diabetic control will help the nervous system to function normally and prevent irreparable damage to the feet.

Warning signs of foot problems may include:

- Pins and needles
- Pain or throbbing
- Swollen feet or ankles
- Red patches on the feet or blueness and blackness of the toes.

Notify your doctor if you are experiencing any difficulties with your feet.

WEIGHT GAIN DURING PREGNANCY

Pregnant women at antenatal clinics are advised that it is normal to put on 28–30 lb (12.5–13.5 kg) during the course of the pregnancy. Some women greatly exceed this figure, whilst others fall far below it without any ill effects on the mother or baby.

After the birth, when the new baby is one week old, it is common for you to weigh 14–16 lb (6.5–7 kg) more than you did before becoming pregnant. Normal weight is generally assumed around three months after birth. Breastfeeding will help to flatten the tummy and reduce the pounds.

The Medical Research Council's Dunn Nutrition Centre in Cambridge is carrying out a detailed investigation into diet during pregnancy. They now challenge the Department of Health's guidelines which suggest that mothers-to-be should eat an extra 250 calories a day on top of the usual 2,100 calories. The study has revealed that individual women's needs vary greatly and that apart from a healthy balanced diet a pregnant woman should follow her appetite.

However, it is difficult for a diabetic woman to follow her appetite. Strict blood-glucose control means that quite often you have to eat when you are not hungry and are unable to eat when you are hungry. The insulin-pen regime does counter the strict timing imposed by two injections of fast- and intermediate-acting insulins, and makes it far easier to 'eat to appetite' during pregnancy without losing good control. Discuss the possibility of using a pen with your doctor.

The rate at which you gain weight during pregnancy is also important. For the first half of pregnancy women normally put on about half a stone (7 lb or 3.5 kg) in weight. For the second half it is usual to gain gradually at the rate of about 1½ lb (0.75 kg) every two weeks. And remember, this is only an average guideline and women should not be apprehensive if they put on much more or much less than this.

It is worthwhile remembering that obesity – being overweight – at any stage during your pregnancy will lower your glucose tolerance, and diabetic instability will increase the risks associated with this.

HUNGER

The natural desire for food for a diabetic is something which can become unnatural in time.

> Recently after lunch with a friend I picked up a couple of items of fruit in order to complete my carbohydrate quota. She commented 'Are you still hungry?' These simple words reminded me of the fact that I hadn't actually felt hungry for weeks. I only ate to order. My diabetic condition has definitely deadened the desire to eat over the years.

Initially when informed I had diabetes, previously unwanted foods became infinitely desirable. Awful items such as stodgy puddings, which I had regarded as disgusting before, suddenly seemed to hold magical treats for me. This period gave way to normal eating, with periods of pigging out on chocolate or sweets every so often. I'm not convinced that a diabetic ever eats normally given the sentence of a lifetime's diet which proves impossible for most people to fulfil.

From my own experience I now have absolutely no interest in food and rarely experience a desire or need for it. Certainly, it is wiser at this stage in your life than at any other to eat a well-balanced diet. During pregnancy banned foods should be resisted and high-quality foods eaten at all times. It is in fact easier to manage this when you are pregnant because the rewards of such good care are so apparent.

Snacks

Women with hunger pangs are often advised to eat sticks of celery and carrot in order to satisfy their hunger but prevent high calorie intake. However, carrots contain sugar and are not a suitable snack for diabetics. Personally, I have never known anyone who has satisfied a craving for food with sticks of celery or carrots, and regard it as a particularly worthless piece of advice. Cottage cheese or any other low-fat cheese with tomato is a more satisfying and nutritious snack, providing protein and yet containing no carbohydrate. A large drink of water, weak tea (contains less caffeine) or low-calorie juice will fill the stomach up and lessen a sudden feeling of hunger.

EXERCISE

Research undertaken on people who exercise has shown that their bodies work more efficiently and that they are generally healthier and less susceptible to colds and flu than those who don't exercise. Diabetics can enjoy all these benefits as well as the important one of reducing the risk of heart disease so prevalent amongst the insulin dependent. Improved overall control is often the benefit of continued exercise. Many people have been able to lower their required insulin dosage considerably after a period of sustained exercise.

If you are unused to strenuous exercise then pregnancy is

not the time to start. However there are exercises you can do which will improve your suppleness and make your heart and lungs stronger, as well as those muscles which will help your body prepare for childbirth.

Fitness is something which should be built up slowly. The golden rules for the pregnant diabetic woman are:

- Don't exercise if you feel unwell or tired.
- Always keep glucose tablets handy.
- If you are going swimming, tell the lifeguard, or whoever, that you have diabetes.
- Wear a bracelet or necklace stating that you have diabetes.
- Stop exercising if you feel pain, are breathless or tired.
- Check your blood-glucose level before you begin.
- Check your blood-glucose level when you have stopped exercising.
- Make sure the clothes and especially the shoes you are wearing are comfortable.

Walking

This is a good way to begin exercising. Try to fit a walk into your daily routine – perhaps a trip to the shops or a short walk after lunch. You should walk at a brisk pace in order to get the maximum benefit.

- Walking will improve your circulation, thereby increasing the flow of oxygen to the baby.
- You will be more energetic as a result of regular walks.
- Walking can easily be fitted into your usual routine.
- Exercising after a meal is a good way of lowering your blood sugar.
- You don't need special clothing apart from a well-fitting pair of shoes.

Swimming

This is one of the best forms of exercise and many women enjoy it when they are pregnant. It will strengthen and tone up the muscles and increase blood circulation. Because it is aerobic (increases the body's consumption of oxygen), swimming will strengthen the cardiovascular system (the heart and blood system) too. Two or three times a week will be enough to make you fitter.

- Swimming will tone up your whole body.
- It is a very enjoyable form of exercise and can be returned to soon after birth.
- You will feel better.

Try not to swim for too long or go too fast – you may not have as much energy as you think. Try to swim with your partner or friend who can watch out for you. Don't swim far out if you are enjoying the sea and remember to wear protective footwear if there is any risk of stepping on coral, sharp stones or other hidden dangers such as sea urchins.

Cycling

Again this is an aerobic exercise. Many people find a home exercise bike a useful way of keeping fit. I used one until I was over seven months' pregnant for an average of 20 minutes a day. I was, however, using it regularly before I became pregnant – I wouldn't recommend this for a pregnant woman who was not fit already.

The advantages of a home exercise bike are that:

- You can wear anything you like.
- You can listen to music, read or watch television while you exercise.
- You can do a few minutes here and there when you have time.
- Your general health will improve as a result.

Jogging

Unless jogging has played a part of your life before pregnancy it is extremely unwise suddenly to take this up when you are pregnant. However, providing you are fit and healthy and have been practising this form of exercise for a considerable time prior to gestation, then it can be continued during pregnancy until it becomes too strenuous or causes discomfort in any way.

- Wear sensible well-fitting shoes.
- Take glucose tablets with you.
- Tell a partner or friend what route you are following and how long you will be.
- Practise a few warm-up exercises before setting off.

- Check your blood-sugar levels before and after the session.

The **advantages** of jogging are that:

- It is an aerobic exercise, which means it will strengthen the heart and circulatory system.
- It can be undertaken easily in any location.
- Continued jogging will aid overall well-being.

Keep-fit sessions

Many health clubs and gymnasiums now offer special keep-fit programmes for pregnant women. Specific exercises to aid the pelvic-floor muscles and general toning up are a good way to prepare the body for childbirth. Ask at your local centre what is on offer.

- Make sure that the instructor is aware of your diabetes.
- Wear comfortable clothes and shoes.
- Keep glucose close by.
- Check your blood-sugar levels before and after each session.
- Only attend classes run by a qualified instructor.

The **advantages** of such keep-fit sessions are that:

- They are adapted to suit the shape of pregnant women.
- The exercises will improve suppleness.
- Specific muscles can be toned up for childbirth.
- They are fun, and a good way to meet other pregnant women.

COPING WITH EVERYDAY LIFE

Many women continue to pursue an active lifestyle throughout pregnancy, even claiming that they have never felt better. For others, fatigue is never far away; for example, morning sickness (often continuing all day) can be very wearisome in the first few months. However the pregnancy affects you, there are some things you can do that will help to avoid the straining of muscles and aid good circulation.

- Bend the knees when stooping to pick up small children or objects. Don't bend forwards from the waist, thereby straining the back.

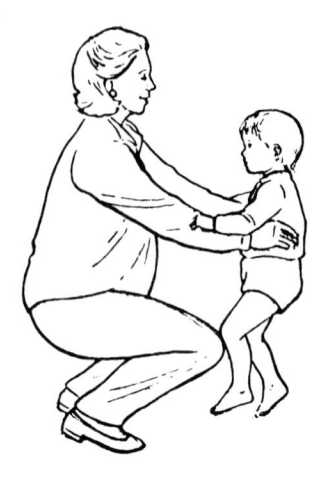

- Try to walk with a straight back when pushing a pram.

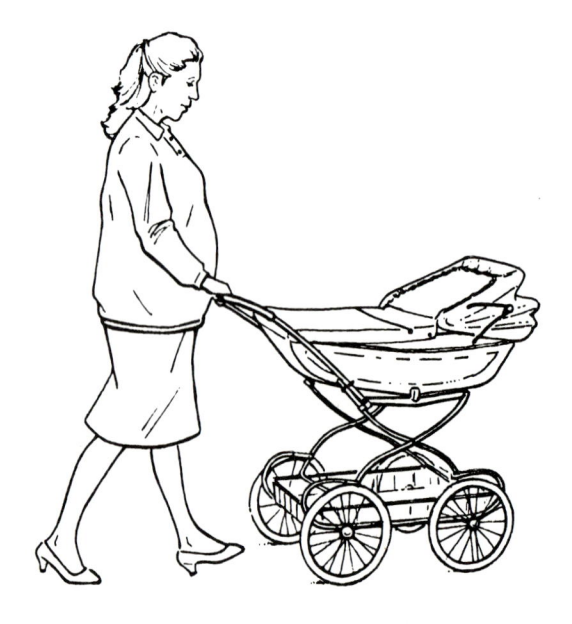

- Carry heavy things close to your body and twist round from the feet rather than from the waist. If possible move the feet and don't twist at all when carrying a weight.

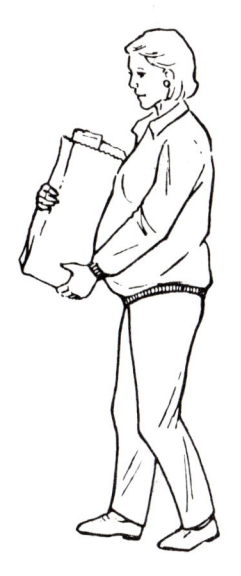

- Turn onto your side before getting out of bed or lying down.

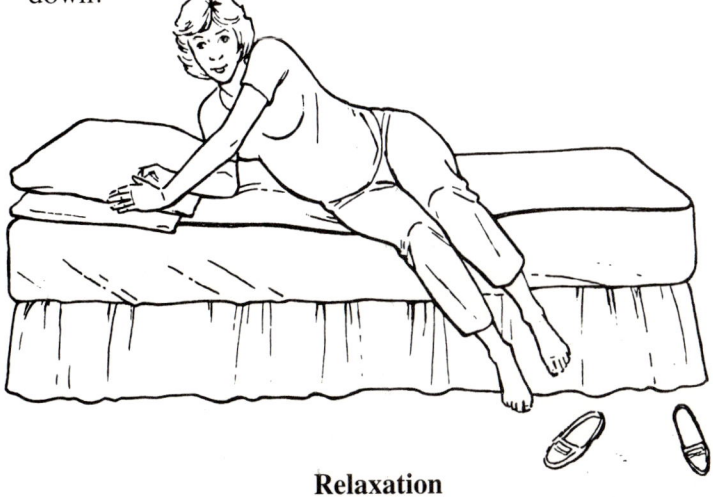

Relaxation

Take a few minutes each day to relax.

- Sit in a comfortable chair with the back supported. Put both feet up in a position higher than your waist so they

are relaxed, or lie flat on the floor with the feet up above your head resting on the wall.
- Lie down and rest on the bed with the head and shoulders supported on several pillows.

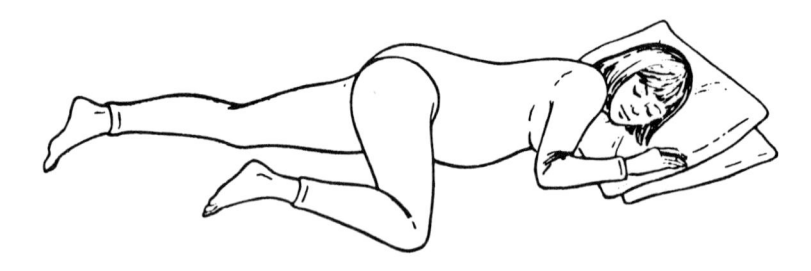

- Lie on your side with your top arm and leg forward and with your other arm and leg behind your body.
- Try not to sit on hard-edged chairs with the legs crossed, as good circulation in the legs is impeded in this position.

EXERCISES EASILY DONE AT HOME

The pelvic tilt

As the uterus enlarges the pelvis tends to tip forwards. This can cause discomfort at best, and extreme backache at worst. To avoid this the pelvis should be tilted backwards.

Stand in an upright posture against a wall. If you do this in front of a mirror you will soon observe if the head, shoulders and body are slouched forward.

- Straighten the neck, tuck the chin in.
- Lift up through the ribs and pull back the shoulders.
- Contract the abdominal muscles to flatten the back against the wall.
- Tuck the buttocks under and tilt the pelvis back.
- Don't press the knees back but bend them slightly to ease the body weight over the feet.
- Try to carry your weight from the centre of each foot.

Pelvic-floor muscles

These exercises were recommended by a specialist well acquainted with the problems caused by prolapsed uteri,

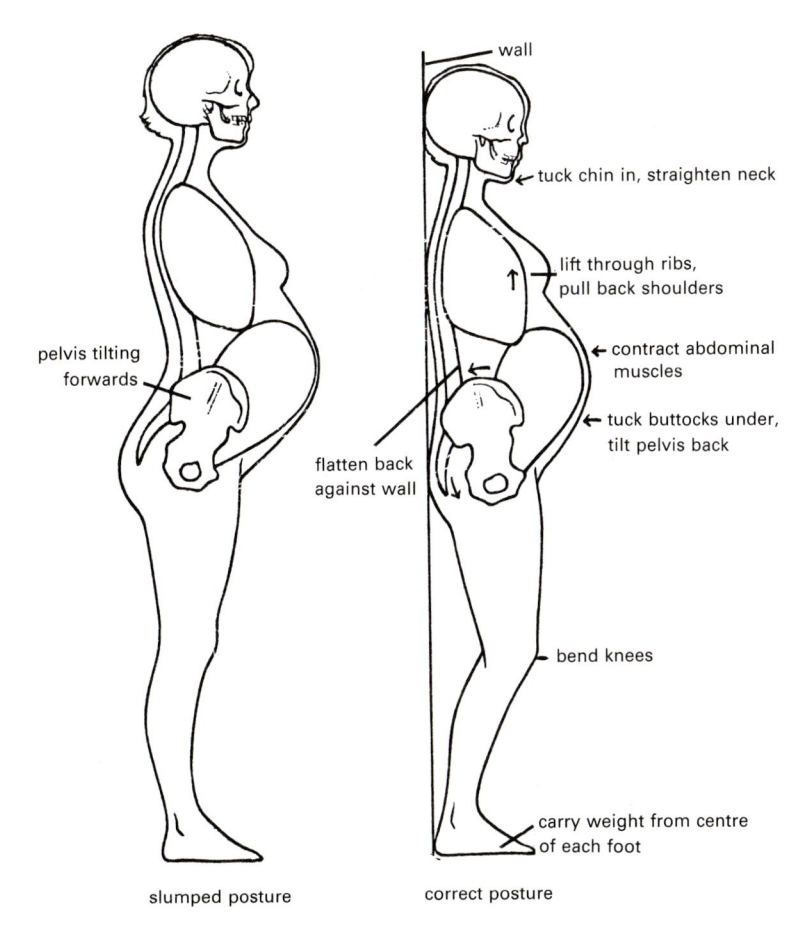

The pelvic tilt.

prolapsed bladders and flabby vaginas.

The same muscles are used in these exercises as in the slowing-down of the flow of urine when sitting on the loo. Identify them by practising stopping and starting when you are peeing. If necessary, use a small hand-mirror to watch the contractions of the muscles as you tighten them.

Once you know which muscles to work on you can contract and relax them anywhere at any time.

- Slowly tighten the muscles in stages until maximum tightness is achieved. Hold and count to five.

- Open the muscles just as slowly and try to bulge them out to achieve maximum width.
- Repeat this five times.

Continue to do this exercise throughout pregnancy, about 10 times a day. Begin the exercises again soon after childbirth – stitches will not be disturbed by them, and the circulation of blood to the area will be increased, aiding the healing process.

Floor sitting

This exercise is often naturally part of the way of life of many Eastern cultures. It will help you to avoid varicose veins and haemorrhoids, as well as improving the circulation in the legs and conveniently supporting the baby during the latter stages of pregnancy.

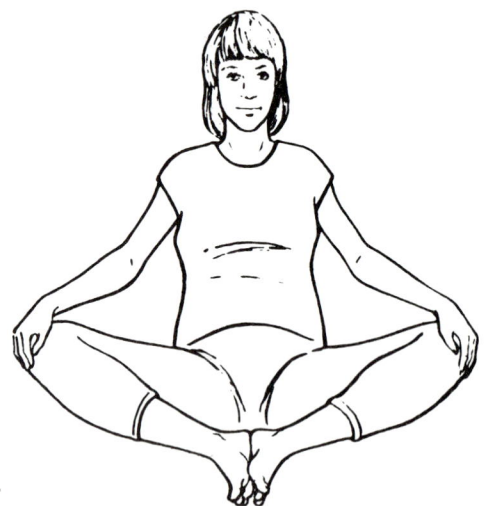

Floor sitting.

- Sit on the floor, with legs stretched out. Bend your knees out at right angles to the body and bring the soles of the feet together, pulling the heels in towards the groin.
- Rest the arms over the legs.
- Keep the back straight.
- Keep the shoulders back.
- Stretch the leg muscles by pressing down gently on the knees.
- Unfurl your legs and stretch them out in front of you.
- Exercise the feet and ankles by rotating them.

AIDS

And as a last word in this chapter, you should remember that AIDS can be spread by:

- Unprotected sexual intercourse.
- A contaminated blood transfusion.
- The sharing of polluted intravenous needles (such as those used in the injection of heroin).

You may be at risk from the disease if you practise or are liable to experience any of these, and if you contract the disease you may pass it on to your unborn baby. However, AIDS cannot be caught or transferred as a result of the diabetic condition.

7

NUTRITION AND PREGNANCY

The doctor and dietitian at the diabetic clinic look very carefully at each diet sheet. Carbohydrate exchange rates are explained and recipes given. I am not going to repeat that information in this chapter – many books on diabetes deal with recommended daily menus in great depth.

Nigel J. Fuller, a research biochemist with the Dunn Clinical Nutrition Centre in Cambridge, has the following advice to offer diabetic pregnant women. Mr Fuller's wife Ann has diabetes and they have a young son.

GENERAL

Lifestyles in Britain have in recent years become more sedentary. The amount of energy needed to maintain this modern lifestyle is therefore less than it used to be, and the food intake necessary to provide this energy has also decreased. The possible danger associated with this is that the intakes of important nutrients may fall as a result of an overall decrease in food intake. In addition, the nutritional quality of some foods is not as high as it might be (too little fresh food and too many convenience foods in the diet). For these and other reasons the food intake of pregnant women may not be ideal.

A healthy varied diet is essential in pregnancy, and your doctor or dietitian should be able to advise you on the most appropriate course of action required to achieve this. If the problem is one of not eating enough, perhaps due to sickness or food fads, small regular snacks may help. Attention to diet is important but should not be obsessive. A well-nourished mother's stores of nutrients in her body should see her over any minor nutritional disturbance. However a healthy varied (balanced) diet should be adopted. Increasing the amounts of starch and fibre and decreasing the amounts of fats in the diet is recommended. Eating much more fruit and vegetables, replacing fatty meats with lean meats or fish, and substituting low-fat alternatives for high-fat products are all possible ways of improving health in pregnancy.

PHYSIOLOGICAL CHANGES AND NUTRITION

Optimum nutrition in pregnancy is that level and balance of nutrient intake which promotes the best health of mother and baby. In the course of a normal pregnancy the growing fetus requires a continuous supply of nutrients from the mother via the placenta, and this demand increases substantially as pregnancy progresses.

Maternal responses to food, or periods of starvation, are modified by the fetus, and by the presence of hormones released from the placenta. The mother's cells become more resistant to the effects of insulin (that is, they are less able to take up glucose) and, as a result, there are changes in her requirements for insulin and balance of nutrients. Morning sickness, lack of appetite (or even increased appetite), food fads (or food intolerance), or just a choice of diet of poor nutritional quality, may adversely affect her nutrition in pregnancy. In turn, this malnutrition of the mother may lead to the birth of infants with low birthweight, impaired mental development and retarded growth.

The fetus and placenta both require a regular supply of energy for optimum growth and development. The current UK recommendations for energy intake during pregnancy are for an extra 240 kcal (calories) per day (1 MJ per day). This represents a 10 per cent increase in the usual energy intake of a non-pregnant woman, and includes the energy needed for the stores of energy-rich fat laid down in the maternal tissues for late pregnancy and lactation.

The period of greatest weight gain in the pregnant mother is between weeks 24 and 32. The extra energy intake needed for this may be obtained from the diet, although surprisingly there is little evidence of this, i.e. pregnant women don't appear to eat more than non-pregnant women. So where does the extra energy come from? Well, a pregnant woman may make extra energy available by altering her pattern of activity and the efficiency with which she carries out her activities. However, the true situation is not clear, and is the subject of much research.

The overall increase in weight during a normal pregnancy is about 26 lb (12 kg) on average, with an acceptable range of about 13–53 lb (6–24 kg). Of this average 26 lb, about 9 lb (4 kg) of fat is deposited in the mother and 1 lb 4 oz (600 g) in the infant at birth; the remaining weight gain is deposited in new tissues (maternal, fetal and placental) and in fluid.

Extra protein is required during pregnancy, for the formation and growth of new tissues in the fetus (1 lb, 400 g) and mother (2 lb, 900 g). An extra intake of protein of about 1 oz (30 g) per day (a 50 per cent increase on the non-pregnant protein intake) is probably sufficient to allow for these added needs, and will be obtainable from a healthy varied diet.

Calorie-controlled diets for slimming must not be taken during pregnancy because they are potentially harmful to the normal development of the fetus. Low-calorie diets, containing low amounts of carbohydrates, may even produce a condition known as ketosis, which can lead to fetal brain damage.

NUTRITION OF THE FETUS

One of the main functions of the placenta is to allow the passage of nutrients from the maternal blood to the fetus. Glucose and amino acids (for building proteins) can be transported across the placenta, even if the mother's blood is low in these nutrients, so that the fetus can still obtain sufficient amounts for its needs. Until recently it was thought that glucose was the only source of energy available to the fetus, but it is now believed that the placenta may also be capable of transporting fats. Some vitamins and minerals also appear to be transported to the fetus, by mechanisms which cause an accelerated uptake towards the end of pregnancy. This sudden heavy demand may considerably deplete maternal stores of iron, calcium and folic acid, possibly affecting the mother's nutrition, unless sufficient stores have been built up during early pregnancy.

The placenta synthesises and releases certain hormones which alter the mother's metabolism, to provide the fetus with its essential nutrients. In generally malnourished mothers it has been shown that the placenta may fail to grow and develop properly. Poor maternal nutrition may also interfere with the synthesis and release of hormones from the placenta. Both of these may interfere with the availability of nutrients to the fetus, and may affect the health of mother and baby. As an aside, the effects of excessive alcohol consumption during pregnancy may cause damage to the placenta as well as to the fetus.

OVERSIZED INFANTS

The birth of oversized infants is a complication of diabetes in pregnancy. Macrosomia, as it is called, is in fact a direct result of poor glycaemic control, and as such is preventable. Maternal hyperglycaemia causes abnormally high levels of glucose to cross the placenta into the fetus, and the fetal pancreas, which starts to function from weeks eight to nine of pregnancy, is stimulated to release insulin in response to this. A combination of high levels of both glucose and insulin causes growth of tissues and storage of excess fats and carbohydrates in the fetus. As well as causing increased growth, severe hyperglycaemia is also believed to be linked with hypoxia (lack of oxygen) in the fetal blood system and fetal death. Furthermore, babies born to mothers with hyperglycaemia during pregnancy may experience a brief hypoglycaemia immediately after birth.

Glucose transfer to the fetus is saturated (that is, no more glucose can cross the placenta even if the maternal levels become much higher) when the maternal blood-glucose levels reach about 11 mmol. What this means is that if maternal glycaemic control is not good it increases the possible risks to the fetus. Good to excellent glycaemic control throughout pregnancy is the best way to achieve a successful outcome.

Improvements in glycaemic control over recent years have lowered the numbers of large babies born to women who were insulin-dependent diabetics before they conceived, but there is still a large incidence of macrosomia in gestational diabetics, in whom glycaemic control is attempted by diet alone. Recent studies have investigated the use of insulin therapy for optimal control of this type of diabetes; it appears that insulin treatment for gestational diabetics actually lowers the rate of macrosomia, and its use is therefore recommended.

DIETARY RECOMMENDATIONS FOR DIABETICS

Apart from the additional amounts required, the quality of nutrition recommended for pregnant diabetics is no different than that recommended for healthy diabetics, and this in turn is no different to that recommended for the population as a whole.

Recent research has led to a revision in the guidelines for what is or is not healthy for a diabetic. It has long been thought that the cornerstone of diabetic control was a low carbohydrate/low insulin regime. However, if the diabetic is prescribed a diet low in carbohydrate, then the extra energy needed for everyday activity is made up by eating fats. Until recently the average energy content of a diabetic diet was composed of 15 per cent protein, 40 per cent carbohydrate and 45 per cent fat. Is this a healthy balance? The answer is probably no; high fat intakes, especially of saturated fats, have been implicated in cardiovascular disease, to which the diabetic is particularly prone. Obesity is another problem to be avoided by the diabetic. In view of these factors, the recommended balance for diabetics (and the population as a whole for that matter) has now been changed to 50 per cent carbohydrate (at least), 35 per cent fat (or less) and about 15 per cent protein.

Are the types of carbohydrate in the diet important? Well, there are two main classes of carbohydrate, simple (sugars) and complex (starches). In normal non-diabetic individuals the simple carbohydrates were assumed to be absorbed quickly into the blood, causing a rapid insulin response. The complex ones were thought to be absorbed more slowly, causing a less rapid response. Only recently has this dogma been tested.

The glycaemic index

The glycaemic index is a useful means of measuring the

relative effects of different carbohydrates on blood-glucose levels. Pure glucose will be absorbed by the bloodstream and will produce an exactly equivalent increase in the blood-glucose level; glucose is therefore given an arbitrary figure of 100 per cent on the glycaemic index. Another carbohydrate may produce only half as big a rise in the blood-glucose level, on a weight for weight basis, when compared to glucose; this will register as 50 per cent on the glycaemic index.

Perhaps surprisingly, it has been found that certain sources of carbohydrate hitherto thought to be in the complex group, e.g. potatoes and bread (white and wholemeal), cause blood-glucose levels to rise almost as rapidly as an equivalent amount of pure glucose, i.e. they may have a glycaemic index approaching about 100 per cent.

Although unrefined foods are beneficial in a number of other ways, the glycaemic response in diabetics should, ideally, be moderated to give blood-glucose levels after a meal of no more than about 8 mmol. Again the emphasis is on a 'balanced' intake. Foods such as potatoes and bread are very nutritious and their consumption is recommended, although, as with everything else, it should be in moderation. However the inclusion of other sources of carbohydrates in the diet of a diabetic, such as those which have a flatter blood-glucose profile (that is, no sudden large peak), is to be encouraged. These foods include rice, pasta, and pulses such as kidney beans and lentils (the glycaemic index may be as low as 40 per cent for beans, while rice and pasta have an intermediate glycaemic index). It should be noted that some foods prepared in different ways, e.g. boiled or baked potatoes and whole or pureed fruits, may also have different blood-glucose profiles.

The physical characteristics of carbohydrates (particle size and so on) may also prove to be important in glycaemic responses. In contrast to the high glycaemic index of some supposedly 'complex' carbohydrates, some simple sugars, for example lactose, fructose, and to some extent sucrose, have been shown to give lower glycaemic responses than might be expected. Some sources of these carbohydrates are not to be recommended because they are energy dense, contributing little other nutritive value (empty calories). However, if they are derived from nutritious foods, e.g. milk or honey, then they can be considered to be part of a healthy varied diet.

Research on the effects of the various carbohydrates on

glycaemic response has, until recently, been concerned mainly mainly with single sources of carbohydrate. It is clear, however, that other foods eaten in conjunction with carbohydrates may modify their pattern of absorption. Proteins and fats (all part of a healthy balanced diet) consumed at the same time as carbohydrates may help to flatten the blood-glucose profile, i.e. slow down the appearance of glucose in the blood. There is also the confounding factor of individual variations in response to various foods. Home glucose monitoring, in addition to attaining good glycaemic control, gives the diabetic the opportunity to judge the glycaemic effects of certain types and combinations of foods for themselves. This enables adjustments to be made in the diet, the aim of which should always be to prevent large fluctuations in blood-glucose levels.

Controversy still exists as to whether or not foods which cause rapid increases in blood glucose are actually harmful or not. If the rise in blood glucose is transient, or if the timing of insulin injections is judged to coincide with it, then it may be argued that little harm is done. Current research is attempting to solve this question, but until a definitive answer is found it is probably wise for diabetics to minimise increases in blood-glucose levels after meals.

Special diabetic foods and sweeteners

Clearly, with the diabetic able to eat a normal healthy diet, the use of special foods is a matter of choice. A high fat intake and excessive use of sweeteners with high calorie value should be avoided. These may limit the intake of other nutrients, or contribute to undesirable weight gains.

Implications for health

There are many potential benefits of these recommended modifications to the diet of diabetics, other than the achievement of tighter glycaemic control. Increasing the proportion of energy available from carbohydrates lessens the need for animal fats. The provision of a greater proportion of fats from vegetable sources as an added measure (remembering that less fat in total is recommended), may improve the ratio of polyunsaturated to saturated fats. Blood levels of cholesterol may also be lowered, and taken together, these changes may reduce the risk of cardiovascular diseases in diabetics.

Changing from refined products to unrefined and fresh foodstuffs will help to increase the intake of dietary fibre, improving colonic (lower gut) function. In addition, it has been suggested that fibre may lower the background glucose levels in normal people. If this is proved to be the case, then fibre-rich diets for diabetics may help with glycaemic control, as well as lowering the amount of insulin required. It may also prove useful in the dietary control of non-insulin dependent (mild) diabetics. Associated with a change to fresher foods will be an increased intake of certain essential vitamins and minerals, which may otherwise be destroyed or removed during the processing of some refined foods.

The use of legumes or pulses (lentils, chick peas, dried beans, etc.) and nuts provides a useful alternative source of protein to that derived from meats and dairy products. The moderate use of lean meats and dairy products as part of a healthy balanced diet is not to be discouraged; some nutrients are more readily available from these sources, for example, iron from meat. Milk is an excellent source of calcium.

WHAT SHOULD I EAT?

What this means is that good nutrition during pregnancy, provided by a well-balanced diet, is vital for the health of the fetus. Furthermore, certain foods will also facilitate good diabetic control and they should form the major part of carbohydrate exchanges.

Carbohydrate

Pasta, lentils and beans are digested by the body more slowly than bread. They should be eaten regularly. The sharp rise in blood-sugar after meals is prevented because of the long-acting quality of these foods.

Protein

Protein is very important for the normal development of the fetus. It also aids the building-up of the uterus and in the formation of breast tissue. Foods which should be eaten daily include low-fat cheese and milk, unsweetened yoghurt, eggs, lean meat such as chicken without the skin, and fish.

Fats and oils

Fats and oils provide essential fatty acids that are needed to ensure healthy fetal development. One of these, linoleic acid, is found in margarine as well as in nuts and seeds. Other essential fats are found in butter, meat and cheese. Higher consumption of unsaturated fats (those which are not of animal origin) is thought to have led to a reduction in the incidence of heart disease in America.

Banned food

Foods which cause blood glucose to rise rapidly should be completely avoided unless they are used in an emergency to remedy hypoglycaemia.

Artificial sweeteners such as saccharine and cyclamates can cross the placenta, and their effect on the baby is not known.

IMPORTANT DIETARY REQUIREMENTS

Calcium

This is a necessary aid for the formation of healthy bones and teeth in the fetus. During the last three months of pregnancy extra calcium is required, as well as phosphorus and vitamins. The recommended daily allowance of calcium for a pregnant woman is 1,200 mg. Foods rich in calcium are cheese, low-fat milk and yoghurt.

Iron

Iron is an essential element in the red blood cells that transport oxygen around the bloodstream, and many women are found to be deficient in iron during pregnancy. Iron supplements are not recommended during the first three months of pregnancy as they can have an adverse effect if not required during this period. However iron is present in high amounts in meat as well as in dried fruits such as prunes and apricots, and in many green vegetables, e.g. spinach or watercress. A diet which included some of these each day will provide the body with all the iron it needs.

Folic acid

Folic acid is essential in the formation of red blood cells, and the body's requirement for folic acid increases considerably during pregnancy. Too little may cause a type of anaemia commonly found in the last three months gestation.

Foods naturally high in folic acid include liver, fresh fruit and fresh green vegetables.

CHANGING HABITS

Try to get your partner and family members to eat more healthy well-balanced meals too. This will help you to stick to your diet. The traditional British diet is high in fat and low in fibre: your diet should ideally consist of the reverse. Your doctor and dietitian will advise you how to calculate the insulin–carbohydrate ratio properly. Always check with them before altering your diet.

A VEGETARIAN DIET

A properly-balanced vegetarian diet is extremely healthy and, if preferred, is to be recommended. However, a change to a vegetarian diet during pregnancy is not recommended; re-educating your body and digestive system to vegetarian ways may take some time and, until such time as a new balance is attained, deficiencies of some nutrients are possible.

Pregnant vegetarians may require additional protein and iron in their diets. Nuts and pulses are good sources of protein, while absorption of iron by the mother, which is increased normally in pregnancy anyhow, may be aided by vitamin C, available from fruits and vegetables (or supplements in cases of deficiency). Vegans run a slight risk of a vitamin B_{12} deficiency, and, if this occurs in pregnancy, may need a supplement.

It remains to be seen whether or not a vegetarian diet is preferable for the health of diabetics. Until then it is a case for individual preference or conscience.

RESEARCH

Current research efforts are being directed towards many aspects of diabetes, and much of this work is concentrated on the benefits and effects of diabetic control and the best ways to attain it. It is felt that some of the complications of diabetes may have a nutritional solution in a better diet combined with proper insulin therapy.

Vitamin C is required for blood-vessel formation and repair, and it is thought that high levels of glucose, as in hyperglycaemia, may interfere with the transport of vitamin C and prevent these processes from working normally. This is currently under investigation. Glucose is also known to attach itself to some proteins, causing extensive damage which may eventually lead to some of the major complications of diabetes. In this respect the development of diabetic complications resembles some of the changes associated with ageing. It is thought that good diabetic control may help to prevent these changes; again, research is attempting to solve this question.

SUMMARY

In summary, it is essential for every diabetic to balance their diet and insulin in order to achieve tight glycaemic control and prevention of large fluctuations in blood glucose. A healthy varied diet is recommended to achieve this. This should be started prior to conception and followed throughout pregnancy, in order to avoid some of the complications associated with diabetic pregnancies.

Diets should be individually tailored, with no hard and fast rules, but with an awareness of what is good and what is bad for diabetics in pregnancy. Individual energy needs should be adequately catered for at each meal, and insulin and meal patterns should be organised to coincide as much as possible. Advice on diet should be available where needed, and, combined with constant monitoring of the pregnancy, should help to achieve the best possible outcome for mother and baby.

Nigel J. Fuller

8

LABOUR

PREPARING FOR HOSPITAL

A few weeks before the baby is due, try to plan ahead for your stay in hospital.

- It can be useful to bring all your insulins and blood-testing equipment with you to the hospital. Everything will then be immediately available to you. The insulin may be taken from you by the nursing staff, and given back at the appropriate times. Safety is one reason for this confiscation; insulin is a dangerous drug if used incorrectly and the nurses can put it in their lockable drugs cupboard.
- Blood-testing equipment can be kept quite safely in the hospital bedside locker by you, and there is no need for staff to appropriate it. It may also be useful for you to be able to test your own blood sugar if you suspect it has risen or fallen, without having to call a nurse.
- Take a few packets of glucose tablets which can be put in an accessible place.
- Sugar-free juices or mineral waters may not be available at the hospital. Bring your own with you.
- Comfortable slippers – a diabetic should wear something on the feet at all times.
- Two or three nightdresses, with front fastenings for easy breastfeeding.
- Maternity bras and pants.
- Dressing gown.
- Super-absorbent sanitary towels. Stick-on ones are easier after birth.

- Daily toiletries – soap, brush, toothpaste and brush, creams and lotions, as well as make-up.
- Money for the telephone – 10 and 50 pence coins.
- Two first-size nappies.
- Clothes to take your baby home in – vest, baby gown, shawl, woolly hat and blanket.
- A large hand-mirror so you can watch the baby's head being born.
- A tape recorder if you wish to listen to music during the birth.

The average length of pregnancy is 40 weeks. However, some women go into labour at 38 weeks and others at 42 and experience a perfectly normal birth.

INDUCTION

Induction is the artificial starting of labour. It is, unfortunately, commonly used to precipitate the birth of a diabetic woman's baby.

Routine delivery of diabetic women at or before 38 weeks gestation cannot be justified on current evidence. If the diabetes is well controlled, the risk of fetal death before term appears to be minimal. Early delivery of these infants, on the other hand, is associated with a higher incidence of the complications of prematurity than occurs in the offspring of non-diabetic women delivered at a comparable gestation, especially respiratory distress syndrome and jaundice.

M.D.G. Gillmer,
Consultant obstetrician and gynaecologist

This view is becoming more and more common.

There may, however, be urgent medical reasons to support an induction before the 38 weeks are up, and certainly many doctors are now inducing around the 38½ weeks gestational time or later.

Advantages of induction

- There can be incidents of sudden unexplained stillbirth in the later stages of a diabetic pregnancy, and many doctors prefer to err on the side of safety.
- There may be medical reasons which make induction necessary in order to ensure the safety of both baby and mother.
- Placental insufficiency. You may be given tests in late pregnancy to check that the placenta is functioning well. The hormone tests check the level of oestriol in the urine or HPL in the blood (see page 25). If the results show that the placenta is not working properly then you may be induced in order to ensure the birth of a healthy baby.

Disadvantages of induction

- Babies born earlier than full term may experience respiratory distress syndrome and other problems.
- The mother may feel cheated at not being allowed to go into labour naturally.
- A possible normal healthy birth may have been interfered with.
- Often failed inductions lead to emergency caesareans with all the attendant complications.

METHODS OF INDUCTION

Prostaglandin pessaries

Prostaglandins are hormones which appear to help the mother go into labour. The pessary is inserted high up in the vagina the evening before the intended birth; the pessary then melts, releasing the prostaglandins.

The **advantages** of this method are that it is:

- Simple to administer.
- No drips are necessary, so allowing you freedom of movement.

The **disadvantage** is that the natural mechanisms enabling the birth process to start have been interfered with.

Artificial rupture of the membranes

This can be performed nearer the expected date than a pessary induction. Alternatively, it is used as an adjunct to a pessary induction if labour has not started by the following day.

A forceps-like tool or a device like a crochet hook is used to puncture the membranes surrounding the baby within the womb, so releasing the waters and inducing contractions, usually within 2–3 hours. At least that is the theory – often it doesn't work, resulting in an oxytocin drip having to be used (see below).

The **advantages** of this method of induction are that:

- It can easily be used when the baby's head is attached to an electronic fetal monitor (see below, pages 90–2).
- The amniotic fluid can be checked for traces of meconium (a substance excreted from the baby's bowels). If meconium is present in the fluid then it can show that the baby is in distress.

The **disadvantages** are that:

- Labour can progress too fast, so being very painful.
- The labour can become too intense; if the cord is around the baby's neck the loss of the cushioning effect of the amniotic fluid can affect the circulation of blood passing through the cord to the baby.

Oxytocin-induced labour

Oxytocin is a natural hormone produced by the body; among other things, it stimulates the onset of labour. Synthetic oxytocin (Syntocinon) can be administered by an intravenous drip to produce the same effect.

The **advantages** of this form of induction are that:

- The use of a drip allows some freedom of movement.
- By adjusting the dose, via the drip, the contractions can be artificially speeded up or slowed down.

However the **disadvantages** are that:

- The contractions can be very strong and as a result very painful.

- As the contractions are often stronger and longer lasting, the periods of rest between them are shorter. This may be detrimental to the baby.
- Many women require the use of painkilling drugs as a result of the stronger contractions which oxytocin induces.
- The success rate is only about 85 per cent.

If you don't want to be induced

Routine induction rates vary from hospital to hospital. Ask your doctor what percentage of diabetic births at your hospital are induced. You may be surprised at the results.

If you decide that induction is something you want to avoid, tell the medical staff long before the expected due date that if the pregnancy is progressing normally for you and the baby and there are no attendant complications due to your diabetes, you would prefer to be left to term. Your doctor may agree with your decision and prefer to leave the pregnancy until labour starts naturally.

If this is not the case and your doctor does not want the pregnancy to start normally, ask him or her what their reasons are. If you are not happy with the answers given, you are entitled by law to change your doctor. The best way to proceed with this course of action is to return to your general practitioner and ask him or her to make an appointment with another diabetic physician or another obstetrician.

LABOUR

False labour

The uterus contracts approximately every 15 to 20 minutes during pregnancy, each contraction lasting about 20–30 seconds. You will probably be unaware of these contractions until the later stages of pregnancy, although occasionally you may be able to feel a hardening of the abdomen.

These Braxton-Hicks' contractions, as they are called, become stronger and occur more regularly in the latter stages of pregnancy, and some women become anxious and convinced that they mean that labour is commencing early. Any concern, such as this, should be discussed with your doctor; otherwise telephone the hospital – they are used to such conversations and will be able to put your mind at rest.

conversations and will be able to put your mind at rest.

Actual labour

Uterine contractions occur every 15 to 20 minutes and, although uncomfortable, aren't very painful to begin with. The duration of these contractions is 40 seconds or more, and they can be timed easily. The passing of blood-stained mucus, known as a 'show', and/or the waters breaking indicate that labour is about to start.

The process of labour follows the same pattern, whether induction has been performed or labour has been allowed to start naturally:

- **Stage 1** covers the beginning of labour through to the full dilation (opening) of the cervix. Dilation can be easily measured by the midwife; when full dilation is reached the cervix is wide enough to allow the baby's head to pass through it – about 10 cm (4 inches).
- **Transition** – this doesn't occur in all births. It marks a brief respite between the contractions of the first and second stages of labour.
- **Stage 2** is the delivery of the baby.
- **Stage 3** takes place after the baby has been born and lasts until the placenta has been delivered.

Length of labour

The average length of labour for a woman having her first baby is 12 hours. Research has shown that forceps delivery and caesarean section are least likely to be the outcome of a short labour. Conversely, the longer the labour, the higher the incidence of fetal distress and delivery by caesarean section.

Women having their second or subsequent babies experience, on average, a labour of six hours' duration. The body is able to perform its task somewhat quicker, perhaps having learned from the first birth just what it is expected to do.

The management of diabetes during labour

Very high blood-glucose levels in the mother during labour causes the baby to be born hypoglycaemic and thereby often necessitates the attentions of the special care baby unit. Normal readings of blood sugar should therefore be maintained throughout labour and caesarean section, and this is the aim of obstetric staff during a diabetic childbirth.

Most diabetic labours are managed with intravenous drips of glucose and insulin in order to prevent hyperglycaemia in the mother. However this form of diabetic management is not mandatory; the drips themselves can actually cause unusually high or low blood-sugar if they are not administered properly or checked regularly, i.e. their use can sometimes result in the very condition they were set up to prevent.

Ask your obstetrician how labour will be managed in your case and what levels of blood glucose are to be aimed for. Prepare your partner to test your blood throughout the labour and get him to write the results down.

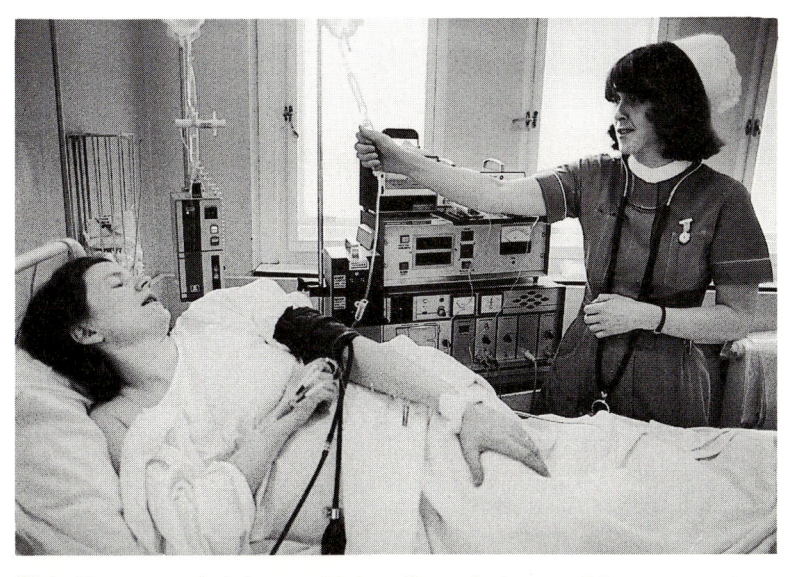

Diabetic woman in labour with insulin and glucose drip.

EPIDURAL ANAESTHETIC

An epidural anaesthetic is an anaesthetic administered to the nerves in the epidural space in the lower part of your spinal column. It has the effect of knocking out the sensations from the lower part of your body. The anaesthetic will be administered by an anaesthetist via a fine tube into the spinal column. The anaesthetist will check its effect throughout labour and top you up if necessary.

An epidural has the advantage of reducing muscular activity in the legs, and so less energy is required by the woman during the labour. I had an epidural for the last seven-and-a-half hours of my twelve-hour labour and it worked exceedingly well. My blood glucose remained at 6 mmol throughout labour without the use of insulin and glucose drips.

The **advantages** of an epidural are that:

- It provides complete pain relief.
- No other anaesthetic is necessary if forceps, vacuum extraction or episiotomy are subsequently needed.
- It can slow labour down, which may be useful in certain instances.
- It lowers blood pressure, making it useful for women suffering with high blood pressure or toxaemia.
- It reduces the amount of energy necessary during labour, making it easier for diabetics to maintain good blood-glucose control.

The **disadvantages** of an epidural are that:

- Episiotomy and forceps delivery are more common, as a result of the mother not being able to feel when to push.
- Some women complain of severe headache after the birth, which may last a few hours.
- If blood pressure in the mother is lowered too much, the oxygen supply to the baby is reduced.
- Not all epidurals are effective for all women.

FETAL MONITORING

The heartbeat of the baby is monitored during labour, either using a fetoscope (which looks something like a trumpet and is placed onto the mother's abdomen and listened through) or an electronic monitor.

Electronic fetal monitoring (EFM)

The fetal heartbeat is usually monitored nowadays using a scalp electrode attached to the baby's head. A belt is also

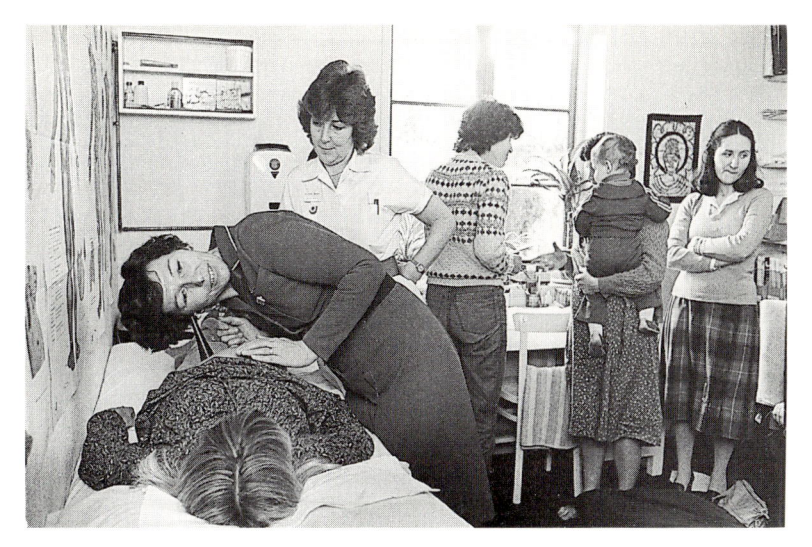

Fetal monitoring using a fetoscope.

strapped around the mother's abdomen to monitor the contractions. In some systems an ultrasound monitor in the belt is used to pick up the fetal heartbeat, instead of a scalp electrode.

The belt and electrode or ultrasound monitor are linked to a machine that gives a continuous reading of the contractions and the baby's heartbeat and allows the midwife and doctors to detect any worrying irregularities or drops in the baby's heartbeat.

Electronic fetal monitoring will be used if:

- Induction is performed.
- Labour is accelerated, i.e. seems to be proceeding too rapidly.
- You have an epidural. With an epidural you often can't feel the contractions, and the midwife and doctors therefore need the monitoring so that they can tell you when to push.
- The pregnancy falls into the high-risk category.

The **advantages** of fetal monitoring are that:

- It indicates when the baby is getting distressed.

- Doctors claim a reduction in the number of stillbirths.
- Doctors also claim it reduces the incidence of mental retardation and brain damage incurred by babies during birth.

There can be **problems** and **disadvantages** too:

- The electrode clip attached to the baby's head can come undone.
- The equipment can fail to work efficiently, giving false readings and so causing unnecessary emergency action to take place.
- EFM restricts the movements of the mother.
- Any small changes recorded may be considered more important than they actually are and intervention may result unnecessarily.
- Three times as many babies who have EFM are delivered by caesarean section, although this is probably a reflection of the fact that EFM will be used in all high-risk pregnancies.
- The clip may be painful to the baby.

EPISIOTOMY

This is a cut made between the vagina and anus (the perineum) to facilitate the delivery of the baby's head. Scissors are used to make the incision, and in theory it should be painless as a local anaesthetic is administered previously.

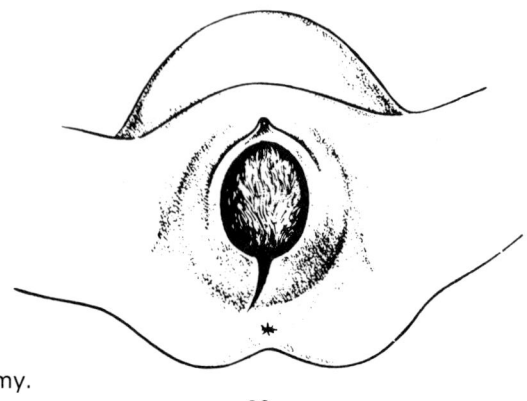

Episiotomy.

Reasons for episiotomy

- If the baby is in an awkward position such as the breech position.
- If forceps need to be used in order to deliver the baby.
- If the baby's head will not pass easily through the vagina and there is a risk of the perineum tearing.
- If exhaustion prevents effective pushing.
- If the baby needs to be delivered quickly, for example if he is suffering any distress.

An epidural anaesthetic increases the possibility of an episiotomy, and as epidurals are a common form of pain relief for diabetic women, you should be prepared for the eventuality of an episiotomy.

Objections to episiotomy

Episiotomy has been blamed for slow healing and painful recovery reported by many women. In addition, women have claimed that:

- An episiotomy is more painful than a tear.
- The subsequent pain after the birth caused discomfort whilst trying to hold and feed the baby.
- Intercourse for the first three months after delivery can be more painful.
- No reasons were given for the episiotomy at the time of birth, so women felt unable to object.
- For some women the damage done by an episiotomy takes years to heal. Long-term problems can be avoided if the episiotomy is performed properly. However, if the incision is made before the perineum has been sufficiently stretched out, excess bleeding may occur, as well as bruising. The pelvic-floor muscles can also be damaged if incorrect stitching takes place, while unnecessarily tight stitches can lead to discomfort during intercourse and surgery may have to be undertaken later to correct this.

How to avoid an episiotomy

- Make sure your medical notes contain details of your desire to avoid an episiotomy unless it is strictly necessary. And

speeding up the birth process without medical reason does not make an episiotomy necessary.
- Make sure the reasons for suggesting an episiotomy are fully explained to you at the time.
- A semi-upright position taken during the second stage of labour will make it easier to have an episiotomy-free birth.
- Learn how to relax the pelvic-floor muscles and use these exercises whenever you can during the birth.
- Try to be aware of the tightening-up sensations of the muscles, so that you can release them at the correct time when the baby's head is being born.

CAESAREAN SECTION

Birth by caesarean section was once the most common method of having a baby available to a diabetic woman. Fortunately, times have changed and vaginal births are becoming more and more routine an option.

However, there are still many varied reasons for performing a caesarean section, and badly-controlled diabetes is one of them. The chances of avoiding a section are reduced considerably if your diabetes is well-balanced throughout the nine months of pregnancy, with very good control achieved during the last two months.

Reasons for caesarean section

Any woman, diabetic or otherwise, is likely to have a caesarean section in the following circumstances:

- Placenta praevia, where the placenta is positioned below the baby's head. This may result in excessive bleeding from the mother's uterus if a normal birth is allowed to occur.
- If labour is prolonged.
- Where induction fails.
- The baby is too large to be delivered normally.
- The baby is presented abnormally in the womb and the positioning cannot be corrected for a vaginal birth to take place.
- As a result of placental insufficiency, i.e. the placenta isn't functioning properly, placing the baby at risk.
- Where the pelvis is too small or malformed.

- If the baby is suffering distress.
- To aid multiple births.
- To prevent the contraction of disease present in the mother (such as genital herpes, where there is a 50 per cent chance the baby will die if it develops it).
- To preserve the health and safety of both mother and baby.

Many diabetic women in fact elect to have a caesarean.

> When I thought about all the equipment they were going to use on me – drips, insulin infusion, inducing hormones, fetal heart monitoring, forceps, epidural, episiotomy (all of which I was told I would have) – I decided that it was not going to be a pleasurable 'natural birth', so I asked for a caesarean under general anaesthetic. This was done the next morning without any problems at all and Laura was born weighing 9 lb 9 oz (4.3 kg). She was observed in special care for 24 hours and was perfect.
>
> *Debbie*

Many women fear that if they have a caesarean section for one baby, then any subsequent births must also be performed in the same way. This is not necessarily the case: a lot of women have proceeded to give birth vaginally after previously having a section.

> I had a good pregnancy with my first child, but was amazed that despite having excellent control and all my scans showing a normal-size baby, they still took me into hospital at 37½ weeks – they kept me in quite unnecessarily, as they left me to look after my own control. The consultant then examined me and despite my having a normal-sized child, they still decided to induce me nine days early, rather than letting me go full term. Consequently my baby was not ready to come and after 18 hours of labour, drips, monitors, etc., he got into distress and they had to do an emergency caesarean. Result – a perfectly healthy baby boy weighing 6 lb (2.7 kg).
>
> I am now on my second pregnancy and have all the signs of another normal-sized baby. Instead of letting them automatically assume I am going to have another caesarean, I have already asked to try to have the child by

normal delivery. I suspect that I will be left till nearer term than the last time.

Andrea

Make sure you understand the reasons given to you for a caesarean section, and if the doctor has not made himself or herself clear, ask again.

Some women are pleased to be offered a caesarean.

I went into hospital at 40 weeks to be induced with pessaries, but wasn't able to get labour started despite three attempts. I was offered a caesarean and took the offer with relief! I had a glucose drip during the operation. My baby son was in special care for 48 hours for the normal blood checks.

Cheryl

How to avoid a caesarean section

- Keep the diabetes in excellent control.
- Keep healthy throughout pregnancy.
- Eat nutritious food with plenty of protein daily.
- Don't smoke or drink.
- Make your feelings known before delivery and during labour. Tell the doctor and midwife that you will only have a caesarean if it is absolutely necessary medically.
- Try to avoid being induced – of the 100 women who wrote to me, the main reason for caesarean section was a failed induction, causing a long labour.

I had a forceps delivery after an induction and 18-hour labour at 38 weeks' pregnancy. I was determined to give birth as normally as possible, though as I lay on the examination table at the antenatal clinic the day I was to be induced, I overheard the doctor mention something about a caesarean section. This is what angers me – they didn't ask me what I thought about it, or even tell me what they intended to do, they were just going to go ahead with it. I piped up and said that unless it was absolutely necessary, I wanted the birth to be as normal as possible, which is why I was so proud once I'd given birth vaginally.

Lesley

Every time I went to the hospital I was praised for how well I was doing, testing my blood sugar three or four times a day. I went for long walks with the dog and kept disgustingly fit, so I was looking forward to a normal delivery.

I was admitted at 38 weeks for an induction. They put a pessary in and told me it would all happen in 24 hours. Nothing happened, not even the slightest labour pain or anything. So next day when I was examined they said the cervix was totally unfavourable as the baby had to be born. I was really upset, after a problem-free pregnancy, not even to have a go at a normal delivery, but I just accepted it and had Paul by caesarean. I had an epidural so saw him come out and that was a great experience. He didn't breathe well, so went to special care for 24 hours. I recovered amazingly well. Eight hours after he was born I was up and down at the special care unit and able to hold him.

Anne

Caesarean and epidural

A caesarean section is performed either using a general anaesthetic or an epidural. If an epidural anaesthetic is used during a caesarean section the patient and partner can watch

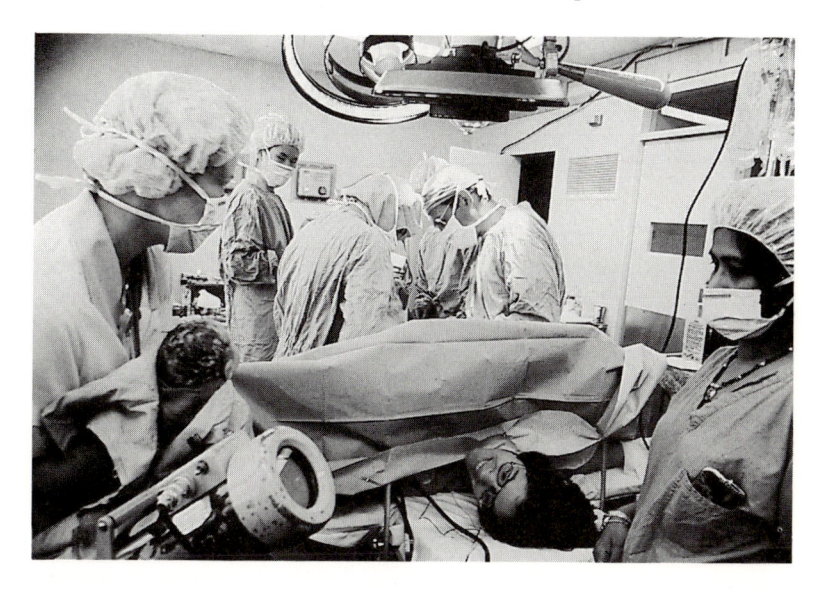

Caesarean birth under an epidural anaesthetic.

the child being born, although a small screen is placed across the abdomen so that the incision does not have to be witnessed. Often the baby is handed to the mother immediately the cord has been cut.

Epidurals have become increasingly popular in the last few years. They allow the mother to be conscious and aware of all that is happening around her, as well as providing complete anaesthesia (lack of sensation) in the lower body.

How to cope with a caesarean

- Try to talk to another woman about her experiences of caesarean section prior to the birth.
- Have your partner with you.
- Get him to take polaroid photographs of the baby immediately after birth so that you can see your infant, even though you may be recovering from the effects of a general anaesthetic and not fully able to get to the nursery or special care.
- Ask the nurses to bring the baby to you as soon as possible.

Ask the doctor how long the scar will take to heal. Ask someone you know who has had a caesarean to show you the scar. Doctors nowadays make the incision below the pubic hairline so that it will not be too noticeable – there is no reason why you won't be able to wear a bikini in the future.

NATURAL CHILDBIRTH

This term refers to birth without the use of drugs or medical intervention. I know of only one occasion that this took place with a diabetic woman – that incident is briefly described in the chapter on gestational diabetes (pages 52–3).

I contacted the well-known natural-childbirth practitioner, Dr Michel Odent, for his views on the subject, with regard to insulin-dependent women, and this was his reply.

> When a woman is an insulin-dependent diabetic, a normal birth, one without any drug or intervention is almost unheard of. The reason for this is the current attitude of obstetrics regarding 'high-risk births' in general, which can

be summed up as reinforcing control. For the mother-to-be, this means going to the maternity ward in advance, or rushing to the hospital as soon as the labour starts. It also means continuous electronic fetal monitoring and assistance from numerous specialised practitioners (midwife, obstetrician, anaesthetist, paediatrician, etc.). The approach leads to an extensive use of drugs, and a cascade of intervention. The more you observe an event which belongs to sexual life, the more you disturb it.

A radically different approach might be proposed, adapted to a society in which most women live less than 20 minutes from a hospital. The theoretical basis for such an approach might be difficult to understand if you have been through a medical training, but is simply this: an easy and fast birth is a safe birth. The primary aim should be to make labour as easy as possible. This implies that 'high-risk mothers' are those who need the best possible environment.

And how can the best possible environment be created? When labour starts, the woman should be able to call *one* very experienced person who will go to her home. Only those people who have the experience of thousands of normal births are able to detect abnormal situations easily, without being intrusive. The woman in labour should be able to behave like any other mammal giving birth, for example hiding herself in a small dark room for a while and feeling free to be noisy and to be in any position. If the first stage is easy and fast, one can choose between staying at home or going to hospital just for the birth itself. If the first stage is long and difficult – a rare occurrence in such a context – this is a good reason for going to hospital. I know from my own experience that this approach works well in cases of a first baby over 40, a vaginal birth after caesarean and a breech baby.

Today it would be logical to take a similar approach in the case of diabetic mothers – nowadays diabetics are treated carefully. When there are no signs of hydramnios (too much liquid) or pre-eclampsia, there is no reason to discourage a vaginal birth at term.

It would be sensible to prepare for the birth with a diet which takes into account the specific needs of a diabetic woman in labour. Cell regulators called prostaglandins are strongly involved in the process of birth. They are made from unsaturated fatty acids. In diabetics, the metabolic pathways of the unsaturated fatty acids are disturbed, so it is a good idea to have a diet high in the unsaturated fatty acids, found in foods such as sunflower, safflower, corn, soy, and evening primrose oil, and in milk and organ meats such as liver and kidneys. On the other hand, it is sensible during the last month of pregnancy to give up eating fish, as fish oils contain fatty acids which inhibit the synthesis of these prostaglandins. (In the Faeroe Islands, where fish is a basic food, many newborn babies are overweight and overdue.) It would also be sensible to supplement the diet with important catalysts such as zinc, vitamin C, vitamins B_3 and B_6 and magnesium.

A physiological birth at term is the best way to prevent respiratory distress of the newborn. It is also the best way to prevent hypoglycaemia in the baby. After a physiological birth it is easier for the baby to consume a good amount of colostrum in the first hours following birth. If there is constant skin-to-skin contact between mother and baby, and unrestricted breastfeeding day and night, some babies do not lose weight at all during the first two days after the birth.

These visions of the future might be considered irrelevant in a book which is intended to inform women about what they are likely to experience at present. But it is thanks to books for lay people written by 'high-risk mothers' that certain attitudes about childbirth are changing. Perhaps the best example of this is an American book about vaginal births after a caesarean (*Silent Knife* by Nancy Cohen). This book helped persuade the American College of Obstetricians and Gynaecologists to modify its previous recommendations.

HOME BIRTHS

I don't know of any diabetic women who have achieved a home birth. However, I am sure the time will come when this will happen. If you want to learn more about home births you can contact the relevant associations which are listed at the back of this book, and discuss your wishes with your midwife and doctor.

POSTNATAL INFECTIONS

A survey carried out by the National Childbirth Trust showed an increased risk of infections of the uterus or of stitches in women whose membranes were ruptured artificially or who had undergone a caesarean section.

To try and prevent such postnatal infections:

- Try to have showers or use a bidet rather than baths.
- Use an alcohol wipe to clean the seat of the loo before you use it.
- When you have been to the loo, wipe yourself from front to back – this will minimise the risk of germs from your anus infecting the sensitive areas after the birth.
- Wash your hands after disposing of sanitary towels, as well as at all other times.
- Bring your own soap to the hospital.

AFTER THE BIRTH

Recovering from childbirth may take some time. Many women find it easier to deal with the postnatal physical problems – extreme tiredness, discomfort, engorged breasts, pain from episiotomy – than the depression which may ensue.

Baby blues and postnatal depression

Around the third or fourth day after birth, when the milk is 'coming in', many women feel weepy and unhappy. Usually these feelings only last a few days and are often referred to as the baby blues. If the unhappiness becomes severe and continues for some weeks then a doctor ought to be consulted, as you may be suffering from what is termed postnatal depression. This condition can strike any new mother, and does not mean that you are in any way unworthy.

9

BREASTFEEDING

A government report published by the Committee on Medical Aspects of Food Policy advises mothers to breastfeed, ideally, for at least a year. They also advocate that:

- All women should be given a chance to discuss their feelings about breastfeeding with a counsellor before birth.
- All babies should be given vitamin supplements until they are at least two years old.
- Women should be allowed to breastfeed immediately after birth and thereafter on demand.
- Complementary bottle feeds should be avoided and free samples of formula milk should not be handed out.
- A mixed diet should be introduced between three and six months whilst also continuing with breastmilk.

Disturbingly, the majority of babies in this country are fed by bottle after only four weeks of age.

Breastmilk is the perfect food for a baby in the first few months of life, and there is no reason why a woman with diabetes should not breastfeed her child for as long as she wants to. I fed my son until he was 21 months old, without any problems. There is in fact some recent research which suggests that women suffering from diabetes are more likely to breastfeed their babies than non-diabetic women. This may be because they are more highly motivated to keep their children healthy by giving them the best possible start in life.

THE ADVANTAGES OF BREASTFEEDING

- Breastmilk has all the nutrients a baby needs.
- Some of the mother's antibodies pass over in the milk, giving the baby some protection against infection.
- Breastmilk is readily available at the right temperature.
- Breastfeeding is relaxing for the mother and baby.
- Both mother and baby can enjoy the close physical contact during breastfeeding.
- Breastfeeding encourages the production of hormones that help the mother's uterus to return quickly to the normal size.
- The metabolic process of milk production and supply improves the general health of the mother after childbirth.
- Breastfeeding is simple and does not involve having to sterilise bottles, measure out formula milk powders and other unnecessary complications.

Colostrum

Colostrum is the first milk a breastfed baby will have. It is rich in protein, minerals and vitamins, and low in fat. It is easily digested by the baby in the first two or three days of life. It also contains concentrated amounts of special substances which will protect your baby from infections such as gastro-enteritis.

Transitional milk

From about the third day, the colostrum changes – it looks thinner and whiter. This milk is just as nourishing as colostrum, but is produced in greater quantity and gives more energy.

This transitional milk, as it comes in, may make your breasts feel overfull, heavy and sore. This is known as engorgement and can be very uncomfortable. In order to relieve the breasts, have a hot bath or sponge the breasts with warm water. This will encourage the milk to flow, so relieving the pressure – and making it easier for the baby to suckle.

HOW TO BREASTFEED

The staff at the hospital, or your midwife, will be pleased to

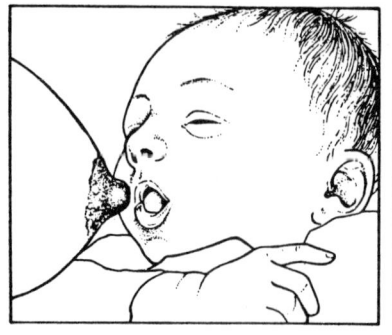

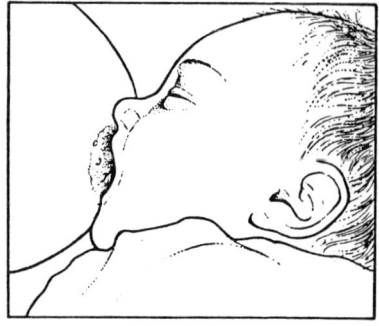

Stroke the baby's cheek so his head is turned towards you and his mouth opened.

Slip in the areola and nipple.

answer any queries or worries you have concerning breastfeeding. Most hospitals actively encourage breastfeeding, so don't be afraid to ask.

- Try to feed your baby soon after delivery. Even if you have had a caesarean section you can still put the baby to the breast.
- To get the baby sufficiently 'latched on', stroke his cheek so his head is turned towards you and his mouth opened. Slip in the areola and nipple.
- Try to sit in a comfortable chair with support for the arms. The baby can then snuggle up whilst being sufficiently supported.
- It is common to feel thirsty just as a feed begins. Some women on insulin may feel their blood sugar going down as the feed progresses. Keep a glass of milk next to you in case this happens. All breastfeeding mothers need to keep up their liquid intake – up to two more pints a day. However, you don't need to drink anything other than water to make up this need for extra fluid.
- To remove the baby from the breast, gently insert a finger between the baby's gums. This breaks the suction so that the nipple slips out without being pulled or bruised.

It is important to remember that the breastmilk produced by the woman with diabetes is just as nutritious as that of the non-diabetic woman. All breastmilk tastes sweet; this is nothing to do with the diabetes.

I breastfed Craig for eight-and-a-half months and am still feeding Carly myself without any real problems. The only thing of course, is watching out for hypos as the breastmilk does take an awful lot of carbohydrate intake.

Linda

How to express breastmilk

Sometimes a baby finds it difficult to feed – the sudden first rush of milk makes it splutter and gulp. If this is the case it may be necessary to express some milk before you start.

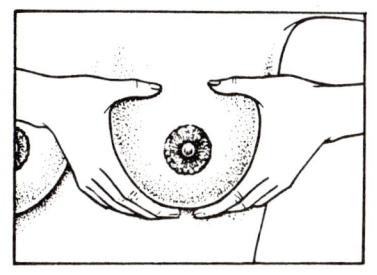

Cup the breast with both hands.

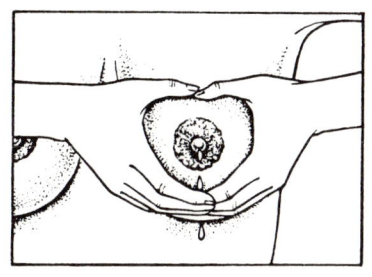

Gently massage the hands towards the nipple.

- Cup the breast with both hands and, by gently stroking, massage the hands towards the nipple. If the breasts are very full then firmer movements may be required. It is easier if the hands are warm.
- Have a sterilised bottle or cup available to catch the milk.
- Keep the milk in a sterilised covered bottle in the fridge, and use within 24 hours.
- Partners can use the bottle of expressed milk to feed the baby, so allowing the mother a little time perhaps for checking her blood glucose.

DIET CONSIDERATIONS

An insulin-dependent breastfeeding mother will require extra portions of carbohydrate without increasing her insulin dosage. An extra 50 grams (2 oz or five portions) a day are the average food increases recommended during feeding. Some women may require more than this, some less. The best way to adjust your diet is by keeping a record of blood sugars before and after each feed and taking these to your doctor at the next clinic visit. Some women decrease their insulin dosage during the breastfeeding period.

> I had to take 22 exchanges while breastfeeding, compared to 18 while pregnant and 14 pre-pregnancy. I found my dietitian invaluable during this time as she was also a breastfeeding counsellor. I fed David for two months and I'm very glad I did, though it was very tiring.
>
> *Maureen*

It may be easier to spread the extra carbohydrate portions throughout the day. Three portions could be made up by taking a pint of milk and two in extra portions of fruit. Of course this extra carbohydrate will not be required when you stop breastfeeding. As the baby is weaned and you breastfeed less, then carbohydrate should be similarly decreased.

> I successfully fed our baby, on demand, until she was nearly 11 months old, when she decided she had had enough. My carbohydrate intake increased to cope with the demand on my body, and gradually my insulin dosage returned to normal.
>
> *Jane*

Hunger

Most mothers feel hungrier whilst breastfeeding, but it is difficult for women with diabetes to satisfy this hunger – blood sugars may rise if too much carbohydrate is eaten. Some women take extra drinks which are low in carbohydrate content, so filling them up and dealing quickly with unexpected hunger pangs between meals. However, if you are markedly hungrier each day, then your carbohydrate allowance may have to be increased to deal with this. Keep a record of blood sugars and tell the doctor when next you visit the clinic.

THE PREMATURE BABY

If a baby is born before its due date it can still be fed successfully by the mother. Quite often premature babies have to be kept in special care for a few days or even weeks. Very early babies may even have to be kept in an incubator.

Breastmilk can be expressed with the aid of a pump and collected in a bottle which is then given to the baby, or the milk can be expressed by hand. Most hospitals have pumps available for mothers to use. As soon as the baby is able to nurse, he can be put to the breast and fed. You will have enough milk if you have been expressing milk every day.

SPECIAL CARE

If the baby is taken into special care for observation for 24 hours, don't be too discouraged. You can still breastfeed. Tell the nurses you want to feed the baby and either ask to be woken and feed your child each time he wakes, or express milk into a bottle.

> I knew Mark would have to go to special care but I asked if I could breastfeed him first, which I did. Although he was there for a week and had trouble absorbing milk at first, and I had a breast abscess at five weeks, I breastfed him until he was a year and a bit old.
>
> *Cathy*

FEEDING AFTER A CAESAREAN

If a caesarean takes place under epidural anaesthetic, which means the mother is fully conscious, then she can hold and feed the baby shortly after delivery. Tell the hospital staff that, should you require a caesarean, this is what you want to do. Providing you or the baby are not in need of urgent medical care, then there should be no reasons for objecting to this.

If the caesarean is performed under a general anaesthetic it may take some time for the mother to recover consciousness and be able to feed. However, if you have a friendly midwife or nurse they can help you hold the baby to the breast.

I did feel upset and disappointed at having a caesarean because it made me feel that Daniel was not yet ready. However, he obviously was. He did have very low blood sugar at birth, mostly, I believe, because my blood sugar rose during the induction. He was fed two hourly and managed to stay out of the special care baby unit. His sugar levels became stable within 24 hours by being fed breastmilk from me and expressed breastmilk from the milk bank until my milk became fully established.

Harriet

BREASTFEEDING TWINS

A mother with diabetes can very easily breastfeed twins, although she may be more tired and have less energy to concentrate on diabetic control. Enough milk will be produced for both babies. It is important, of course, to eat regular well-balanced meals. Extra carbohydrate other than the 50 g already mentioned may be required. The dietitian will look closely at your daily needs with you.

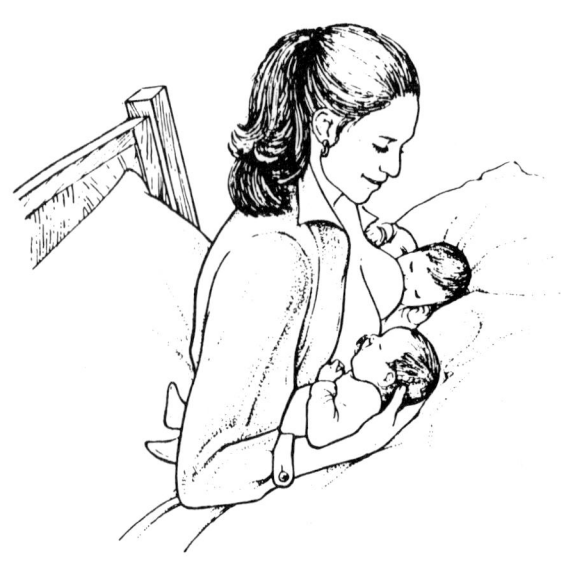

Breastfeeding twins.

After an anxious start I ended up feeding my twins for much longer than I expected (18 and 21 months). Despite various problems I did not need to use bottles at all, nor did I start them on solids until they were five-and-a-half months.

Sue

Extra help may be required if you have twins. Try to enlist that help before getting home from the hospital. Try to eat well, and take some rest whenever you can.

PROBLEMS ASSOCIATED WITH BREASTFEEDING

Inverted nipples

If the nipple fails to become erect when the baby tries to latch on, or he cannot grasp the nipple properly in order to feed, a plastic or glass breast-shield may help to draw the nipple out. Some hand or electric breast-pumps work well, and you can put the baby to the breast immediately after using the pump.

The alternative is to express the milk into a bottle and feed the baby this way. Many women have been able to breastfeed successfully with inverted or flat nipples.

Sore and cracked nipples

Sore nipples are caused by the baby biting on the base of the nipple instead of closing on the areola. Babies suck quite vigorously, so once the nipple is in the mouth, direct it upwards towards the roof of the mouth. Some of the areola should be in the baby's mouth as well. If the baby's chin is touching the breast then the gums should be correctly pressing on the areola, not the nipple.

Washing the nipples with soap can make them dry, so try to avoid this. Alternating breasts with each feed will stop one nipple getting an unfair share of pressure. Some mothers find a rubber nipple shield helpful, as it acts as a screen to protect your skin but allows the baby to suckle normally.

Mastitis

This is an infection of the breast which can develop from a cracked nipple or a blocked duct. Once an infection has developed it may take a long time to heal because the infection may interfere with diabetic control. Any sore spots or lumps in the breast should be reported to the doctor or midwife immediately, so they can be dealt with promptly.

Babies with abnormalities

Some handicapped babies are unable to breastfeed successfully. Babies with a physical problem, such as a hare lip and cleft palate, may not latch on properly, so are sometimes unable to feed. However, the baby can still be given the mother's milk if it is first expressed into a bottle.

Demand feeding

It is impossible to say at what times of the day or night your baby will be hungry, which is why it is best to offer the breast whenever you think it may be needed. Most babies stop crying when they are fed – the desire for physical contact and cuddling may be as great a need as the demand for milk.

Some babies will suck for what seems like hours, whereas others will suck for short amounts of time, perhaps more frequently. Or the baby may do both of these things, at different stages. Frequent suckling does stimulate the milk supply, so the more the baby feeds, the more milk the mother will have available. Constant suckling is not a sign of insufficient milk.

It is best to be as flexible as the baby's needs require. If she wants to feed, take the opportunity to put your feet up and relax.

Nightfeeding

Almost all small babies wake up at night, whether they are breast or bottle-fed, and often they continue to wake up like this for weeks or months.

Keep the baby close to you at night so that feeding is simple. Either have the cot next to the bed or sleep with the baby. I found it easier to take our son to bed. When he woke he rested on my arm and helped himself. I found this to be the easiest and least disturbing method of coping with nightfeeding. However, some mothers and their partners prefer the baby in a cot next to the bed, in which case the baby can be easily picked up, fed and put back, without too much activity.

It is easier to keep a glass of milk by the bed in case your blood sugar falls too low during a nightfeed. You could also have some glucose tablets to hand on a table next to you; if the baby is in bed with you, glucose tablets kept routinely under the pillow may be furred out by the baby. My bedside table was pushed as close to the bed as possible, so that all that was required was a languid stretch of the arm. Extra drinks close by help night thirsts when breastfeeding, and low-calorie juices or water won't affect carbohydrate exchanges.

REASONS FOR STOPPING BREASTFEEDING

Research has shown that women with diabetes stop breastfeeding for exactly the same reasons as any other women.

- Lack of milk
- Baby not sucking properly
- Sore nipples
- Illness of mother or baby
- Baby self-weaned
- The mother wanted to stop

BREASTFEEDING – A MOTHER'S EXPERIENCE

The following account by a diabetic mother of how she breastfed her three children first appeared in the diabetic's magazine *Balance*. It is reproduced here by kind permission of the British Diabetic Association.

> I have been an insulin-dependent diabetic since 1960 and my first baby, William, was born in 1976 when I was 28; the second, Alice in 1978; and the third, Chloe, in April 1981 when I was 33. I do not intend to have any more, though we would if I were not diabetic.
> I fed William until he was 17 months old and Alice until she was 22 months. I am now feeding Chloe (who will soon be six months old) about four times in 24 hours. Once out of the maternity hospital I never used a bottle.
> Before William was born I was in a state of blissful ignorance – I had seen my mother feed a brother 10 years younger than myself so 'knew how to do it' and I intended to feed my baby myself. When I mentioned at the antenatal classes that I was diabetic I got a rather vague and

discouraging response: 'I don't think they always allow diabetics to breastfeed.' This made me very determined to do so.

William was induced at 37½ weeks, weighing 8 lb 10 oz (3.9 kg) and had a forceps delivery because he became distressed and took a long time to breathe. After a short cuddle he went to the special care baby unit for three days, during which time I had no contact with him at all. They had an infection in the main unit and William and other younger babies were in a side ward off the labour ward and no mothers were allowed in. We could only look through a glass panel in the door.

This was an unhappy time for me, and had I read then what I've subsequently read about bonding, etc., I would have been worried. I rather timidly mentioned to the SCBU sister that I wanted to breastfeed; she was surprised but not discouraging. On day four I was called down to feed William. By this time I was full of milk and luckily he turned out to have a talent for sucking and all went well. It was explained to me that he would have to be test-weighed because if he did not get sufficient calories, his blood sugar might fall too low. If he had not taken enough milk he was to have a top-up bottle. I soon found that if I attempted to feed him four-hourly, as required in Hull Maternity Hospital at that period, he would not feed properly if woken up to feed and took very little. Test-weighing would show that he'd not had enough and I'd give him a couple of ounces from a bottle.

This made me angry so I declared UDI and fed him only when he woke up to be fed – quite irregularly – sometimes after two hours, sometimes after six. Test-weighing then showed that he was getting a lot of milk from me and we were both discharged on day six.

Being more experienced when Alice was born, I told the baby unit before she arrived that I would breastfeed her. She arrived normally at 38 weeks, weighing 8 lb 2 oz (3.7 kg), but her blood sugar fell rapidly after birth and only rose after she'd had a drip in her scalp. She was also tube-fed through the nose until the SCBU sister thought I was likely to have enough milk. At that point, day three, I moved from the postnatal ward to a little room attached to the SCBU. I was not asked to test-weigh Alice, nor was I expected to top her up with a bottle, although the same sister was in charge. Again, with Alice being tube fed in an incubator, I had not been able to hold her, apart from briefly after delivery, until I fed her on day three. I was able to go and visit her at any time and to touch her through the holes in the side of the incubator. We were discharged on day five.

Chloe was induced at 37½ weeks and arrived after a very quick and easy birth, weighing 8 lb 9 oz (3.9 kg). After delivery we had a long cuddle; my husband was present at both her and Alice's birth and sent out for William's. She started rooting for the breast and sucked avidly for some minutes. About an hour passed before she went to the baby unit. It turned out, once she was there, that her blood sugar had fallen very low indeed and she drank an enormous quantity of milk from a bottle. This restored her blood sugar to normal but she continued to be very greedy. She lost about 7 oz (200 grams) in the first few days.

I had no stitches and felt very fit and confident and was able to spend a lot of time in the baby unit. I would be called at feeding times (except at night, at first) and would breastfeed and then bottle-feed Chloe, until my milk came in. She was never in an incubator. She came up to the postnatal ward on day three but to my surprise I found it much more difficult to feed her. I fed on demand for the first day on the ward and she went back to the unit at night. That first night she became 'twitchy' and had to be given something to restore her blood sugar. This made me nervous and I felt I had to top her up with a bottle in case this happened again. The sister from the baby unit was encouraging. She made me realise I would never leave the hospital if I were anxiously to send Chloe back to the baby unit every night so that she could be watched for signs of twitchiness.

I stopped complementary feeding and fed Chloe very frequently for about 36 hours. Her blood sugar remained gratifyingly high and we were discharged on day six. She has remained a greedy child and is much larger now than were either of the other two at this age. She did not slim off after birth as diabetics' babies are supposed to do and as the other two did. She weighed 16 lb (7.3 kg) at five months.

I have dwelt at great length on my period in hospital with

all three because I feel that this is the most difficult time for a diabetic mother. You are anxious to get home and you know that neither you nor the baby will be discharged until your diabetes is reasonably stable and the baby's blood sugar remains constantly high enough. Add to this any worries about having enough milk, etc., and I can see that many mothers might be tempted to give up and bottle-feed. This would be a great mistake because, once established, breastfeeding is so easy and such a lovely experience.

I have always fed on demand but have found that they have settled down to some kind of routine quite quickly. Such a routine does change, of course, even over the months. By the time they were three or four months old, all of mine wanted to be fed at mealtimes – before they were on solid food – but I find it easy enough to feed myself and the baby at the same time. I am careful about what I eat and like to eat at regular intervals and have not found that demand feeding interfered much with my routine. You don't have to feed a baby for very long to satisfy it for a while. You can do almost anything while feeding a baby if you want to – answer the telephone, wipe a three-year-old's bottom, etc!

It was never suggested to me that I should alter my carbohydrate intake while breastfeeding until Chloe was born, but I found with the first two that I had cravings, which I indulged freely in calorie-rich food such as butter, cheese and peanut butter. With my third I have eaten more carbohydrate – about 40 g a day more – and less fat and find that a more satisfactory arrangement. In five-and-a-half months I have gradually lost about 6 lb (2.7 kg) in weight. After Chloe's birth I had put on about 7 lb (3.2 kg). I am not a stable diabetic – I alter my insulin frequently and test my blood sugar four times a day. I have three injections a day. I have not found that breastfeeding has made me any more or less stable, while exercise or lack of exercise has a marked effect on my insulin needs.

I have never paid any attention to people who might say things like 'Maybe she's crying because your milk's too thin/ not enough/too thick/too sweet/not sweet enough/been affected by swimming in the sea/climbing a mountain/eating curry/grapes/cabbages/oranges, etc.' I feel that until they can prove to me that such statements are true they are worthless, or worse, because they could be so discouraging.

When Alice had just cut a tooth at six months she bit me and the tiny cut became sore and a little infected. An antibiotic cream from the doctor cured that quickly. I was much more worried to find that when Chloe was about six weeks old I developed what the family doctor described as an 'incipient breast abscess'. There was no obvious cause but I had an increasingly painful breast for about a week and it did not drain properly when Chloe was sucking. I went to the doctor and the condition cleared up slowly with a five-day course of antibiotics. I have had no trouble since. I continued to feed both babies throughout and neither showed any ill effects.

Another difficulty diabetic mothers may face is the attitude of staff at the infant welfare clinic. Not all health visitors are aware that a diabetic's baby may be born unnaturally fat and is likely to slim off or gain weight rather slowly at first. As I have said before, this has not happened with Chloe. When surrounded by other mothers whose babies gain 8 oz (225 g) a week, a 2 oz (50g) weight gain by a breastfed baby tends to raise some eyebrows, and makes the mother feel defensive. I feel that as long as your baby is reasonably happy, healthy and gaining a little weight fairly steadily you should not worry. I have found that I knew more about diabetes and about the expected weight pattern of my babies than did the clinic staff. It is a good idea to discuss this with the paediatrician before you leave hospital and then you can speak with some authority.

Susan Palfremans

10

THE BABY

Most babies born to women with diabetes are extremely healthy. The importance of good blood-glucose control prior to conception has already been stressed; the continuation of that control during pregnancy is also imperative. If you find you are pregnant and have not been very careful about testing your blood sugar, it does not automatically follow that the baby will suffer any problems. Strict control will, however, improve the chances of having a perfect baby.

THE BABY AND DIABETES

It is extremely rare for a baby to be born with diabetes. The infant of a woman with diabetes is, however, more likely to be born with low blood sugar than that of a non-diabetic mother.

The fetus of an insulin-dependent mother may have had to deal with larger-than-normal amounts of sugar crossing the placenta during pregnancy. The baby's pancreas is working normally by that stage and, in order to cope with the extra amount of glucose, it produces a larger amount of insulin than usual so that the fetus' own blood-sugar levels can be kept within normal limits. Once the baby is born and the umbilical cord is cut, this supply of sugar from the mother stops. The baby's pancreas may continue to secrete extra amounts of insulin though, and the baby's blood sugar falls, causing an insulin reaction. If the mother keeps her own blood glucose balanced during labour, the extra sugar will not be crossing the placenta continually and this reaction will not occur.

The baby's blood glucose will be checked by the hospital,

especially during the first four to six hours of life, when symptoms of low blood sugar may appear. Breastfeeding soon after delivery – I fed Jackson a few minutes after birth – helps combat the effects of low blood sugar. Some babies are given intravenous glucose and water soon after birth if the glucose reading is very low initially.

Usually special monitoring is required for only the first 24 hours, by which time the baby should be tolerating feeds well. Hypoglycaemia rarely occurs after the first few days of life, so, providing the baby is feeding well and frequently, this should not cause concern.

Heredity in diabetes

Research has shown that the children of parents with diabetes have a 1–5 per cent chance of developing the disease. Research has also shown that children whose parents both have the disease are more likely to develop it than the child who has only one parent with diabetes. It has also been shown that children are more likely to develop the disease if the father has diabetes rather than the mother.

SPECIAL CARE

'Nowadays less than 20 per cent of babies require admission to special care, most for observation alone' (Dr M.D.G. Gillmer).

Not all babies born to women with diabetes require the initial 24 hours of special care. Many women ask and are allowed to keep their babies with them and feed them on demand, just like any other mother. Check with your hospital what routine they follow and let them know what you would like to see happen with your baby. Some babies, however, do require the facilities of special care for a longer period.

I have recently given birth to a son, Lee Adam, on 13 January. I had a trouble-free pregnancy, although it does take some effort and perseverance to keep it that way. However, being impatient like his mother, he decided to arrive seven weeks early. He was not really due until 3 March. Mind you, he was a reasonable size considering I was only 33 weeks, even with all my strict and pretty good control.

I was told originally that I would be induced at 38–9 weeks, but as things went that didn't happen. I had a normal delivery (no forceps, etc.) after a short labour of only nine hours. As for Lee, he was in the special care baby unit for three weeks and we are more than grateful for the care they gave him. He has recently been given the all clear by the hospital and is now thriving like any five-month-old.

Mrs A.I.

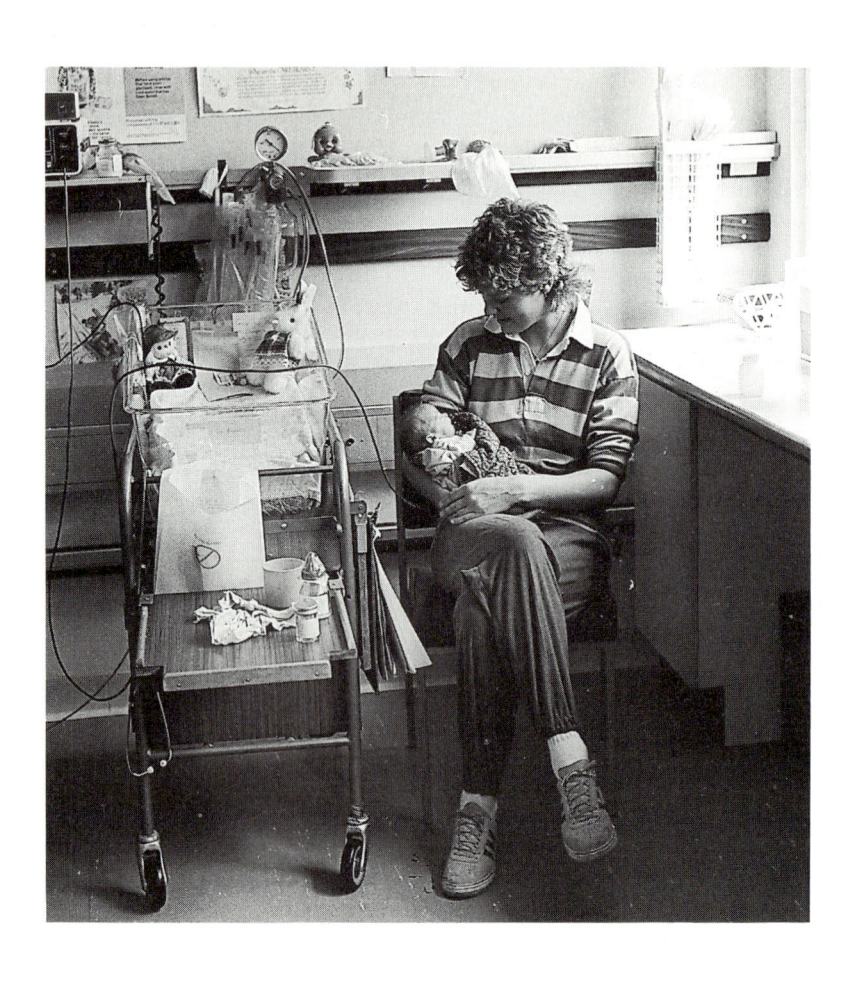

The special care baby unit.

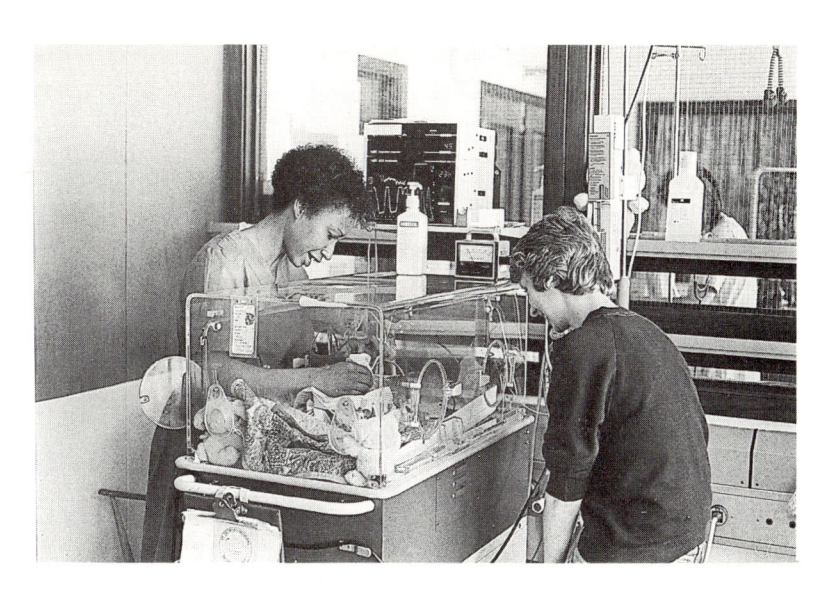

Incubator care.

I was pleased that my babies were admitted to the special care baby unit. The special care here is small and informal, allowing mums to live in there or stay with their babies for as long as they like. I appreciated the knowledge that the nurses are more aware of the circumstances of diabetic pregnancies and babies of diabetics.

Linda

A real advantage of special care was the extra time staff had to help with feeding.

Jane

PROBLEMS ASSOCIATED WITH BABIES OF DIABETICS

Hypocalcaemia

Some babies are born with a low blood-calcium level; this happens more often to babies of women on insulin. The symptoms are similar to those of hypoglycaemia and are easily treated by an intravenous infusion of calcium. No serious problems result from this condition, and parents should not worry about it.

Jaundice

This is due to a breakdown of red blood cells in the fetus. A byproduct of this breakdown is bilirubin, which is dealt with by the liver and excreted in the bile. The liver of the new-born baby does not deal with the bilirubin efficiently and it becomes laid down in fat beneath the skin, so causing the skin to have a yellow tinge. Sixty per cent of all infants suffer a degree of jaundice.

Most mild forms clear up untreated after a few days, but if the level of jaundice is very high, the baby may be treated with phototherapy. The infant is placed under an intense light source which breaks down the bilirubin in the tissues just beneath the skin into a form which can be readily excreted by the kidneys.

Respiratory difficulties

Some babies born of women with diabetes suffer from breathing problems in the first few hours or days of life. These difficulties can be dealt with by oxygen treatment for a short time.

Babies with breathing problems are much less common now than they once were, due to better control during pregnancy and better means of fetal assessment.

Macrosomia

A baby with macrosomia is heavy and obese at birth. Usually a baby is born in this condition if the mother's diabetes has been poorly controlled during pregnancy.

Abnormalities

The general population runs a slight risk of infant abnormality, to the order of 1 per cent. With women who have diabetes this rises to just under 4 per cent. Most abnormalities can, however, be treated.

Every pregnant woman spends some time during her pregnancy worrying about giving birth to a baby with some sort of abnormality. I think it is reassuring to know that these statistics on abnormalities existed before the routine use of blood-glucose monitoring strips, so with better control during pregnancy the percentage must fall further, in line with that of other women.

I was horrified to hear the list of possible problems linked with diabetes in pregnancy. I had a lot of help and support from my GP and diabetic consultant. My pregnancy was quite normal and Sam was 6 lb 13 oz (3.1 kg) at birth.

Christine

TWINS

The chances of a woman having twins can be determined by a genetic counsellor quite easily. The likelihood increases if there are twins in the family and if a woman has a large amount of children. Twins are also more likely to be born if a woman has had *in vitro* fertilisation, or has been taking fertility drugs. These same rules apply to a woman with diabetes; she is no more, or no less, likely to bear twins than anyone else.

The nutritional demands on the mother carrying twins are greater than on the mother bearing one baby, and it may be difficult for some women to meet these demands by sticking to a normal diet. It is because of this that twins are frequently born prematurely, quite often by caesarean section.

SUDDEN UNEXPLAINED STILLBIRTH

Mortality rates of babies born to women on insulin have been steadily falling each year. Hopefully this is due to increased care during pregnancy. 'As a result of major advances in obstetric diabetic and neonatal care, the majority of pregnancies of diabetic women now have a successful outcome' (Dr Judith Steele). With this comment in mind it is perhaps easier to read the following tale.

I have been diabetic since the age of three years. When I was 21 I started to become almost insulin resistant and developed severe complications to my diabetes, but fortunately I recovered from most of them as my control improved.

When we married in 1978 I was warned not to leave it too long before we tried for a family as I might have some difficulty in conceiving. We left it for a year and in July 1979 I found I was pregnant. I was admitted to hospital for assessment and fortnightly for the next six months I spent a night in hospital for blood-sugar series to be done, despite the fact I had my own glucose meter. I felt my home blood sugars were surely a better reflection of my control than the ones where I spent 24 hours on my bed. However, all went well until 36 weeks of pregnancy, when I suddenly started having severe hypos without warning. I was admitted to hospital as they thought there was something wrong with the baby or that the placenta was failing, causing my blood sugars to drop. I spent the next week having intravenous glucose and minimal insulin and finally at 38 weeks they decided to induce me. The baby eventually became distressed and an emergency caesarean was performed. Our first son Oliver was born weighing 7 lb 8 oz (3.4 kg) – a delight to us, as deep in my mind I never believed we would have children.

Our second son Dominic was born on 31 December 1982, again by caesarean section. He was a big boy, weighing 9 lb 1 oz (4.1 kg). I fell in love with him instantly. This time I had still been admitted fortnightly in late pregnancy as my blood sugars were much higher this time and my insulin requirements were greatly increased. But all was well, thank goodness, and now he is a fine healthy bouncing four year old.

I love children but never thought of planning any more, even though I would have liked a larger family. The diabetic physician said two children were enough for a diabetic and I was lucky to have them, so we didn't think we would have any more.

Then in May last year, despite having had a coil fitted, I found I was pregnant. There was both delight and trepidation; delight because I didn't think I would have any more children, and trepidation because I had not controlled my diabetes particularly well prior to conceiving. However, as soon as the pregnancy was confirmed I went straight to the diabetic clinic, and from there started the old routine of testing my blood sugar four times daily, going through the hypos, the worry, but I went through it all for our bonus baby!

Because it was so difficult to keep my blood sugars at a reasonable level, I was changed from two- to three- then ultimately four-times-daily insulin and spent three days in hospital for this. But that was all the time I spent in hospital whilst I was pregnant. It was decided the caesarean would be performed on January 2 or 9, depending on my control. On the 31 December I went for my last antenatal visit and all was well. It was arranged that I be admitted on the 8 January for an elective caesarean under epidural.

On Tuesday 6 January the baby stopped moving. I phoned my GP, but the receptionist told me that this was quite normal towards the end of pregnancy. On Wednesday I was still worried, so I phoned the GP again. He came, but could not hear the fetal heart. When we arrived at the hospital the consultant was waiting for us. A scan was performed which showed the baby had died and we all assumed it was due to the diabetes.

The obstetric consultant was wonderful, so kind. It was decided that I should have a caesarean as soon as possible. When they performed the section they found the cord had ruptured spontaneously and our beautiful daughter had died because her blood supply had been cut off. You can imagine how devastated I am. Life goes on, and has to for the sake of our two sons, but the pain I have to bear is constant.

Through the diabetic pregnancy network you set up I have been in touch with other mothers who have also lost children. It has been a help to hear from them. Although every baby is special, a diabetic mother's baby is an extra special baby because, whatever anyone says, it is through the mother's co-operation and hard work that a healthy baby can be produced. I know what happened to me could have happened to anyone. My consultant said he had only seen it happen once in 10 years, and that time was to a non-diabetic woman.

Carmel

How to cope with a stillbirth

- Ask the nurses or your partner to take a photograph of the baby. This has often helped women with their grieving and serves as a precious momento to many.
- Try to see your baby. This will help you deal with the death and may prevent fantasies about the baby's looks haunting you in the future.

- Talk about the death and your feelings to friends and relatives. People are often afraid and embarrassed to bring the subject up.
- Hospitals often make all the funeral arrangements in these circumstances, and this has sometimes caused deep distress when parents learn that their baby has no identifiable grave or headstone. Parents can decide on the kind of funeral they want for their baby and make these arrangements themselves if they so choose.

11

MANAGING THE BABY AND YOUR DIABETES

HOSPITAL STAY

Mothers now stay in hospital for about five days with a first baby; this period is often less with a subsequent baby. A woman with diabetes who has been given a caesarean section may have to remain in hospital for a week or longer, so take all your insulin and sugar-testing equipment with you when you pack your bag for the hospital. All that you need will then be instantly available. Put a couple of packets of glucose tablets in an accessible place as well.

As soon as the baby is born your insulin requirements will return to pre-pregnancy levels, and the dosage may be further reduced if you are breastfeeding and experiencing a few hypos. Keep a note of your sugar levels whilst in hospital.

It is easy at this stage to forget about your diabetes, especially when you have produced a bouncing healthy baby. Tiredness and overwhelming delight can take its toll on your energy levels. Added to this, the recovery period needed for an episiotomy or caesarean section can all too easily be ignored, especially if your baby is alert and wakeful and wanting to be fed often.

ARRIVING HOME

Throughout the nine-month gestational period women become fixated with the birth, unable to imagine life after it and often feeling that the event itself is akin to throwing a dice and hoping it lands on a six.

Some women experience the natural low of an anti-climax once the birth and all its attendant furore has subsided; and life as you knew it previously may be considerably altered for quite some time after the birth. As a friend of mine recently remarked:

> The birth of our baby has affected every area of my life, including relationships with other people and the relationship between my husband and myself. My once neat and tidy home is a complete disorganised mess, I feel tired permanently and just long to stay in bed for most of the day!

The community midwife will visit you and your baby at home until the tenth day after birth, and the health visitor will then take over. Both the midwife and health visitor are there to assist you; make sure you have their phone numbers readily available and don't be afraid to contact them if anything is bothering you between visits. They are specifically trained to help you through your first few weeks; make sure they are fully conversant with your diabetes and tell them how it affects you.

BE ORGANISED

Try to arrange for a partner, friend or relative to help for the first couple of weeks at home. A clear division of labour is sometimes helpful; many women want to spend their time with the baby and find a helpful mate is useful if he or she does all the shopping, washing, clearing up and cooking.

Organise the home so all the baby things are in one place. Put the pram or crib next to a comfortable chair suitable for breastfeeding, so that the baby can easily be laid down when he falls asleep. Put the phone next to the chair so that you don't have to dash off to answer it in the middle of a feed. Alternatively, take the phone off the hook and grab some time to relax and put your feet up each time you sit down to feed. Keep some glucose tablets and water within reaching distance – quite often when you just sit down to relax you find you are amazingly thirsty. The breastfeeding woman requires a great deal of extra fluid and it can be infuriating to have to get up from your seat to get yourself a drink.

SLEEPING

For the first few weeks, or even months, the baby may sleep and wake erratically, perhaps only sleeping for two hours at a time in the first few weeks. This can be physically exhausting and you may feel inclined to drop off for an hour or so at the same time.

However, if your insulin regime consists of one or two injections a day, then the danger of sleeping through the set eating time is obvious. A doze just before lunch, or a few minutes sleep after having an injection and before eating, can be very dangerous. It is best to make it a rule never to do this without first checking your blood-glucose level, or asking a partner or friend to wake you at the appointed time. Quite often, however, you will be on your own with the baby, in which case keep all your insulin equipment near the chair where you will be breastfeeding.

If the insulin regime consists of a few insulin injections a day, at varied times using an insulin pen, then more flexibility is allowed. It is then easier to fall asleep when you are tired, even if it does delay your next injection; a little long-acting insulin will still be floating around your system, so there is less likelihood of unexpected severe hypos if the diabetes is well controlled.

RUNNING THE HOUSE

Nothing quite prepares you for the complete exhaustion of the first few months if your baby is lively and healthy and if you are feeding on demand. However, life can be made easier.

- Try to get a partner, neighbour, friend or relative to do all your shopping in bulk.
- Get disposable nappies delivered to the home if you can.
- If friends ask if you need any help, show them where the ironing board is kept and talk to them while they work.
- Set a few hours a week aside for housework and try not to get upset when you do get surrounded by a mess.
- Sit down as often as possible.
- Make the time to eat properly – plenty of fresh fruit, protein, vegetables and high-fibre carbohydrates.

- When people drop in unexpectedly, get them to make the tea – most people are only too happy to be of use.

MEALTIMES

One or two injections a day, consisting of a mixture of short- and long-acting insulins, require rigidly-timed meals. The temptation may be to grab something sweet, such as a few biscuits, and so avoid a hypo and deal with the sudden influx into the system of insulin. No doubt on a few occasions, when things are very hectic, this will happen. However, it is important to eat well-balanced meals so that you feel well and produce nutritious milk for your baby.

Sometimes the appointed lunchtime hour may occur, you are just about to sit down and eat . . . and the gasman arrives to fix the central heating, the baby spills his juice all over the washing, your grandmother phones in the throes of a heart attack, the washing machine floods, etc. Honesty is normally the best policy in these situations – explain to whoever is there that you have diabetes and you must eat now, then leave all domestic matters until you have eaten. The mess won't have gone away, but you will probably be better able to deal with it. At the very least, have a small glass of fruit juice – enough to get you through the crisis – and then return to your meal.

Insulin pen injections consist of a short-acting insulin which is given half an hour before a meal. There is a small amount of long-acting insulin in your system, given conventionally at night, but this acts as background insulin and does not provide the peaks needed for meals. Obviously, on this regime, meals can be planned to take place at less crucial times if a busy day is expected, or a meal and an injection can be missed out altogether without any problems. However, a domestic crisis can just as easily occur between an injection and a meal. In this case some carbohydrate should be taken if the meal is going to be longer than 40 minutes after an injection. And if you are about to have an injection when an emergency occurs, then simply delay the insulin and meal until you have dealt with it. No harm will occur if eating and injecting are delayed for an hour or two.

If the baby settles down for a long feed just as you are about to eat, make certain you have some cheese sandwiches or natural yoghurt handy so that you can eat whilst breastfeeding and without fear of spilling anything hot on to the child. It is certainly inadvisable to drink anything hot with a baby on your lap.

POSTNATAL DEPRESSION

Many women think they are experiencing the beginnings of postnatal depression when they feel shaky, tired and prone to crying for no reason on or around the third day after giving birth. Quite often these symptoms are just part of having the 'baby blues', and disappear a few days later.

For some women, however, the symptoms of extreme anxiety and depression linger, and these can become impossible for the new mother to deal with on her own. Women with diabetes or any other disease are just as likely (or unlikely) to suffer from postnatal depression as any other mother.

Most doctors can be very sympathetic and aware of all the problems postnatal depression presents, once the diagnosis has been made. If you feel you might be suffering from severe depression after the birth of the baby, tell your health visitor. They will be on the lookout for it and will not be surprised by your feelings.

And remember that suffering from postnatal depression does not mean that you are not a good, loving, caring mother.

ISOLATION

You may feel quite lonely once the initial euphoria has subsided and the daily demands overwhelm you. Now is the time to get out and talk to other people. If you don't have friends with small babies, ask your health visitor if she knows of any playgroups or mother-and-toddler groups. A lot of women bring tiny babies to these groups for the company they provide and also the stimulating effect small children have on babies.

If you have not made contact with any mums with diabetes, phone the Care Department at the British Diabetic Association and ask for details of the network. Go to coffee mornings in your area arranged by the National Childbirth Trust organisers. Find out what is available locally by asking other mothers.

COPING WITH THE DIABETES

Should I inject in front of my children?
Very often a woman with diabetes has no choice but to inject in front of her children; sometimes it is unsafe to leave a child in a room on his own. It is very difficult to do anything which requires privacy when you have very small children.

I have always tested my blood glucose and injected in front of my son, and as he becomes older so he has shown more curiosity in what I'm doing. I have made it quite clear that these are mummy's things and that he is not allowed to touch them. When he is a little older I will explain quite carefully what each item is for.

However, all insulins, syringes and blood-testing equipment, including all spares, must be kept in a safe place, at all times, out of children's reach. It is best to choose a lockable cupboard and always remember to put things away. Of course this can be immensely inconvenient at times, but insulin is a dangerous drug and must not be misused.

Glucose tablets
Some parents give their children glucose tablets as a form of sweet; as such tablets are usually readily available in the home of someone with diabetes, this is an easy enough thing to do. However, a problem can arise when the child has eaten all the glucose tablets and the adult with diabetes cannot find any when having a hypo.

Saving time
With small children in the house, time is often at a premium. For example, people with diabetes spend a lot of time visiting their general practitioners with requests for insulin, syringes, blood-glucose strips. This is often because the prescription given at the end of a diabetic clinic visit does not last until the next clinic appointment. If it is necessary to get such top-up or repeat prescriptions from your GP, it is often easier to post your list of necessary items to the doctor, along with a self-addressed envelope in which the prescription can be returned.

Most doctors are quite happy to go along with this form of request, and it saves unnecessary journeys.

When you have deposited the prescription at the chemist, tell him you will be back in half an hour and go and do the shopping. Don't wait for the chemist to make up the prescription, otherwise you will have to entertain a baby in a busy shop.

And ensure that you are well equipped with supplies of insulin, etc., after your baby is born, enough to last for the first couple of months.

Safety and needles
You can obtain a clipping device which cuts off the point of the needle, on prescription from your doctor. This will enable you to dispose of your syringes safely.

Travelling
Whether you are going away for a few days or a few months, always check you have your insulin and other apparatus before leaving the house. Once, when I was moving house, I managed to have my insulin packed by the removal firm who were clearing up before loading the contents of the kitchen onto the van. This meant a last-minute dash to my doctors by my husband for a prescription, plus a visit to an obliging chemist who remained open to complete the request. I now have two complete sets of insulin and syringes, which I keep in different places.

Long-distance journeys by air can be a nuisance for the person with diabetes.

- Ask the stewardesses the times of all meals and snacks before departure.
- Don't be afraid to test your blood sugar whilst seated – sometimes it's impossible to get to the loo.
- Give a small injection of short-acting insulin before each meal and leave the long-acting insulin until you arrive and resume your normal activity.
- Keep a spare set of insulin, syringes, glucose and blood-testing equipment in your handbag at all times.

A DIARY

I kept a diary throughout my pregnancy and some of the notes I made after the birth make quite entertaining reading now. It certainly reminds me of how hectic life can be initially with a new baby.

Jackson 10 days old. The days seem to slip by and I no longer know whether it's Tuesday or Wednesday. In fact it's Saturday. Jackson is getting more and more beautiful.

Jackson 13 days old. I'm absolutely exhausted. I got up at 4 am and was awake all morning. He wanted to feed and feed all night. I just couldn't settle him. I managed to have a bath and lunch, then Jackson wanted another feed. I fell into bed at 12.30 until 3. Dave took over, keeping Jackson with him while he worked – Jackson only slept for half an hour however. We all actually had supper at the same time in the evening.

Jackson 16 days old. I am surviving on a maximum of five hours sleep a day, in two separate sessions. I can't remember what a night's sleep feels like. At least Jackson is thriving. Dave and I look extremely ill.

Jackson 20 days old. We all ended up watching a film recorded previously on the video at 4 am this morning. Managed one-and-a-half hours' sleep later, before lunch, despite the barking dog next door which drove me completely wild. We all went for a walk before tea. It was nice to see a bit of the world. — came round and recounted all the latest trivia. We both found this very boring compared to the endless fascination that Jackson provides.

Jackson four weeks old. One whole month today. The days are still totally merged into each other. Spent all day in my nightie. Jackson hardly slept at all and was grizzly. I gave him two baths in an effort to get him to sleep, but this seemed to charge him up instead of settle him down. When did I last wash my hair? I am only testing my sugar now at crucial times – Is it low? Is it high? I can't manage it before meals.

12

SEX AND CONTRACEPTION

There is no evidence to suggest that the sexuality and libido of a woman with diabetes is any different to that of any other woman. And there is no reason why an insulin-dependent woman should not have a full and enjoyable sex life.

SEX DURING PREGNANCY

Sexual intercourse during pregnancy does not harm the fetus as the penis does not penetrate the womb. Unless there are particular medical problems, sexual intercourse during pregnancy can be as enjoyable as at any other time.

Comfortable intercourse during pregnancy
Often pregnancy provides a situation which encourages couples to be more inventive in their sex lives, especially in the latter stages. As Sheila Kitzinger points out, couples may need to be more flexible in their responses:

> If pregnancy is advanced, it may be better for the husband to ejaculate just before the woman enters the phase of accelerated rhythmic movement that results in orgasm. This may seem odd advice when books stress that the man must wait, but she may be unable to embark on free movement of her pelvis and the pelvic-floor musculature when the penis is still erect and rigid inside her. Thus hampered in her movements, the chances of her reaching orgasm are reduced. So it may be best for the husband to ejaculate first, and then with caresses (or otherwise) to lead his wife onward to her own orgasm.

Recommended positions for lovemaking whilst pregnant

- Lying on the side with the partner lying behind. The vagina is entered from the rear, so allowing the woman some freedom of movement.

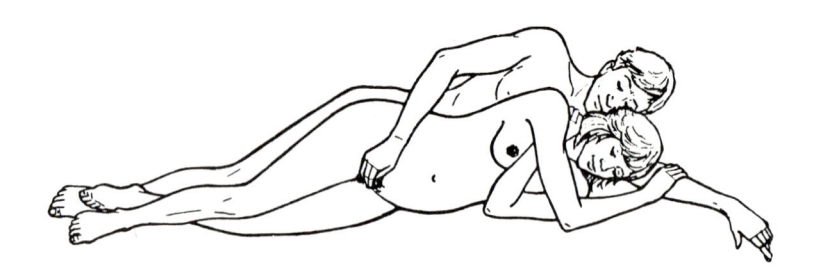

- Woman sitting on top. With this position there is deep penetration, but the woman can control it.

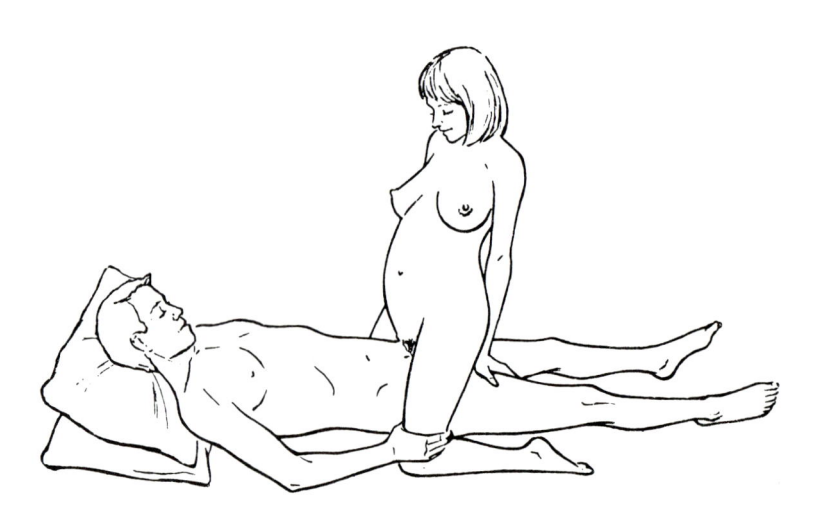

- The woman kneels and leans on the bed, with her partner behind. This is a comfortable position for late pregnancy.

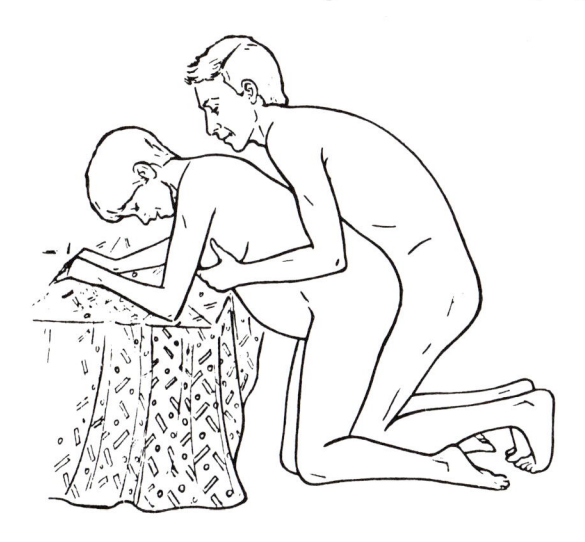

Discomfort
The breasts may be tender and feel full during pregnancy. Some women report a heightened sexual pleasure, whilst others feel uncomfortable. Women sometimes worry that sex can cause a baby to miscarry and this unfounded fear can lessen their sexual desire.

Whatever the concern, talk to the doctor about it. He or she will be able to reassure you.

Desire
Some women notice a lessening of desire for sex during pregnancy, thought to be because of changes in the hormones circulating in the body. Cuddling, stroking and caressing may be just as satisfying during this time.

When should I stop having sex?
A full sexual relationship can continue until the waters break.

SEX AFTER CHILDBIRTH

Masters and Johnson in their book *Human Sexuality* report that women are usually fit for sexual intercourse a week after giving birth. Some women would vehemently refute this, especially if they are still suffering after a caesarean section or an episiotomy or simply from general exhaustion.

The best time to resume your sex life is when you and your partner are ready. This may not be for weeks, or even months, after giving birth.

BLOOD-SUGAR CONTROL AND SEX

Some women notice a lowering of blood-glucose levels after sex and keep glucose tablets close to the bedside or under the pillow. Make sure that your partner can recognise the symptoms of low blood sugar.

It may be advisable to raise the level of carbohydrate before going to bed at night. The added exhaustion of sleepless nights and very busy days, once the baby has been born, may mean that sex will lower the blood glucose at night even further.

CONTRACEPTION

The best time to consider contraception is immediately after the birth. Even though sex may be the last thing on your mind, you may not have time to consider it when you are rushing around at home seeing to the baby's needs as well as your own.

Contraceptive advice will be given at the first check-up six weeks after giving birth. It is important not to miss this appointment. Keeping a supply of condoms in the home is the easiest way of dealing with the initial few weeks until the first appointment, at which point other methods of contraception can be considered.

Full breastfeeding

Hormones produced during breastfeeding delay the onset of ovulation; breastfeeding can thus act as a natural form of contraception. The **advantages** are that it:

- Is easy to use.
- Requires little planning.

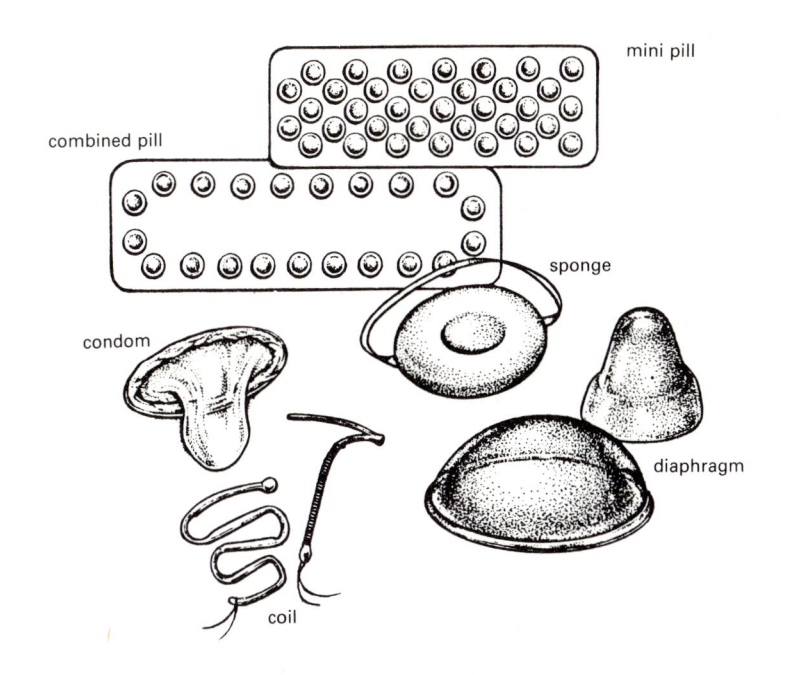

Contraception should be considered immediately after the birth.

However, the **disadvantages** are that:

- It cannot be relied on as it doesn't work for everyone.
- It is not so effective if the baby is only partially breastfed.

The combined pill

This consists of a combination of progestogen and oestrogen, and is almost 100 per cent effective. It shouldn't require you to alter your diabetic control, although some women do need more insulin whilst taking this type of pill. Its **advantages** are that:

- It is simple to take.
- Some people suffer no side effects.
- It is more suitable for the younger diabetic and for the short term.

Its **disadvantages** are that:

- It cannot be used if you are breastfeeding as it can suppress your milk supply.
- The risk of heart disease is increased. As diabetics have a higher-than-average risk of heart disease anyway, this makes this type of pill even more inadvisable.
- Vomiting and/or diarrhoea can mean the loss of protection – other contraception should be used until the next period.
- It is therefore not suitable for the older diabetic or for long-term use.

The mini pill

This consists of progestogen only, and is about 98 per cent effective. The **advantages** are that:

- It is simple to take.
- There are less risks associated with it than with the combined pill.
- It is recommended by doctors for diabetics of any age.
- It does not alter your diabetic control.

There are **disadvantages** though:

- It is not quite as effective as the combined pill.
- Irregular bleeding or spotting can occur.
- As with the combined pill, vomiting or diarrhoea can mean the loss of protection, and other methods of contraception should be used until the next period.

The coil

The coil or IUCD (intra-uterine contraceptive device) is 96–8 per cent effective. Its **advantages** are that it:

- Is easily fitted by a doctor.
- Does not require a daily routine.

However its **disadvantages** are that there:

- Is a high risk of failure.
- Can be complications if a pregnancy results when a coil is in place.

- May be an increased risk of infection for diabetic women.
- Can be irregular bleeding.

It is therefore not always recommended for diabetic women.

The condom
This method can be 97 per cent effective if used with a spermicidal cream. Its **advantages** are that:

- It is simple to use once you get the hang of it.
- It has a high protection rate if used properly.
- It only needs to be used when required.
- There are no health risks – in fact there are positive advantages as it offer high protection against AIDS and cervical cancer.

The only **disadvantages** are that it:

- Can interfere with lovemaking.
- Can cause embarrassment.
- Can burst.

Overall, therefore, it can be recommended for diabetics.

The diaphragm
As with the condom, this method is 97 per cent effective if used with a spermicidal cream. The **advantages** are that:

- It is simple to use.
- You only need to use it when required.
- There are no health risks.
- It offers some protection against cervical cancer and AIDS.
- It gives a high protection rate if used properly.

The **disadvantages** are that:

- It can be messy.
- Some men say they can feel it.
- You've got to remember to remove it.
- It must be checked regularly for holes and tears.
- It needs to be refitted after childbirth or after a loss or gain of weight.

As with the condom, it can be recommended for diabetics.

The morning-after pill

This consists of a high dose of oestrogen. Its **advantage** is that it can be taken within 48 hours of unplanned sexual intercourse or rape. However there are a number of **disadvantages**:

- It can only be prescribed by doctors – it is not available over the counter at chemists.
- Close follow-up is required after taking it.
- It is certainly not recommended as normal routine contraception.

The sponge

This is reputed to be 85 per cent efficient, although research varies as to its effectiveness. Its **advantages** are that:

- It is simple to use.
- It provides protection for 24 hours after it has been inserted.

Its major **disadvantage** is that it is not very effective.

Injectable contraception

This is a relatively new method of contraception, consisting of a long-acting injected dose of progestogen. It is almost 100 per cent effective. There are a number of **advantages**:

- It is very effective – there is no possibility of forgetting to use it.
- Each injection gives three months' protection.
- There are fewer side effects than with the combined pill.

One of the **disadvantages** is that it can disrupt the menstrual cycle. Furthermore, the guidelines produced for the use of this contraceptive state that it should be used with extra care on women who are diabetic.

As this method becomes more widely used, then more research into its advantages and disadvantages will become available. As yet, however, it is still in its infancy.

Coitus interruptus
If a couple are not too concerned about a pregnancy occurring, then this method could be practised happily, providing the diabetic control of the woman was good (in case she did get pregnant). The obvious disadvantage of the method is its high failure rate. Furthermore, it imposes an abnormal strain on the man.

Sterilisation
This method can only be considered once a couple have completed their family, but it is 100 per cent effective – this is its great advantage. However, if the woman is to be sterilised it does require a general anaesthetic. And, very rarely, pregnancies have been known to occur afterwards, sometimes years after the operation to either the man or the woman.

This method is sometimes the preferred option for diabetic women and their partners.

NATURAL FAMILY PLANNING

This works by a couple not making love during the fertile days of each menstrual cycle and is rated as 85–93 per cent effective. There are various methods of calculating when these fertile days occur.

The Billings or mucus method
The woman has to keep a close watch on her cervical secretions – wetness is a sign that ovulation is about to occur. To prevent conception it is therefore recommended that sex is avoided when wet mucus appears and whilst it lasts, as well as for four dry days afterwards.

The temperature method
A strict record is kept of the body temperature each day, in order to detect a slight fall and then a noticeable increase. This sudden change indicates that ovulation has occurred. Making love is then avoided from the first day of a period until three days after ovulation.

The calendar method
A woman notes the dates of her period over six months to a

year. The pattern of her cycle can then be assessed and the likely days of fertility worked out. This method has a high failure rate and isn't recommended, as ovulation can occur over a number of days in the menstrual cycle and it varies considerably between women, therefore making an accurate calculation very difficult.

Your doctor will advise you in detail on natural family planning. It can have a high failure rate and requires a great deal of motivation and effort. Paradoxically, many couples practise these methods in order to find out when to conceive, rather than to prevent conception.

ABORTION

Diabetic women are able to, and sometimes do, terminate their pregnancies. Diabetes, in itself, is not a sufficient reason for ending a pregnancy, although it may be considered if there are other indications which also support an abortion.

    A glucose and insulin drip will be attached before you are given a general anaesthetic, although a lot of early abortions are now carried out under local anaesthetic and do not require loss of consciousness or an overnight stay in hospital. Make sure, in either case, that you have someone with you at home for a couple of days following the operation and keep a careful eye on blood-glucose levels, so that control can be easily maintained.

    Recent research by the Royal Colleges of Obstetricians, Gynaecologists and General Practitioners into the long-term consequences of abortion has found that women who have terminated their pregnancies are no more likely to suffer illness in the next pregnancy, or have babies with birth defects, than any other women.

13

QUICK QUESTIONS AND ANSWERS

THE BABY

How many diabetic women have healthy babies?
Over 90 per cent of diabetic women give birth to healthy babies.

Will my baby be born diabetic?
This is extremely rare. However, he may be born suffering from low blood sugar as a direct result of your diabetes. This can easily be treated.

Will my child develop diabetes?
Not necessarily so. If you are insulin dependent the chance of your child developing it is less than one in 10.

I have twins – will they become diabetic?
If you have identical twins and one develops juvenile-onset diabetes, the other twin has a 50 per cent chance of developing it too. However, that does not mean that because you have twins they are more likely to become diabetic.

Will my baby automatically be put in special care?
No, unless the baby is born with very low blood sugar or other problems and needs careful monitoring. Some hospitals have a policy of non-separation from the mother, except in cases of emergency. State your preferences, before the birth.

How many children can I have?
Many doctors recommend that a diabetic woman limits herself

to two children so that both the demands of the children and the diabetes can be adequaely met. However, if you wish to have more children then medically there is no reason why you shouldn't.

If I have a hypo will my baby suffer?
Research has shown that unborn babies tolerate low blood sugar remarkably well, if they are infrequent. They do not react so well to very high blood sugar.

Can I breastfeed?
Yes. Most diabetic women prefer to breastfeed as they know it is the best possible food for their babies. Extra carbohydrate should be taken to maintain good control.

THE HOSPITAL

Will I have to spend long periods in hospital during pregnancy?
No. If your diabetes is well controlled throughout pregnancy there is no need to spend any time in hospital.

How long will I stay in hospital when the baby is born?
The average hospital confinement for a first baby is now five days. Some women, however, manage to go home after six hours, whereas others have to wait a few weeks. If all is well you will be able to leave at the usual time.

Will my partner be able to attend the birth?
Yes. There is no reason why the birth of a baby born to a woman with diabetes should be treated any differently in this respect.

Will lots of medical people be present at the birth?
The midwife, a nurse and an obstetrician may be present at the birth. Your permission will be asked if other medical staff want to attend, apart from the diabetic physician. They will be perfectly understanding if you say no.

CAESAREAN SECTION

Must I have a caesarean?
Some women elect to have a caesarean section. Your doctor will decide if a caesarean is absolutely necessary. More and more diabetic women are now giving birth vaginally, though.

I had a caesarean last time – will I have another one this time?
No, not necessarily. Many diabetic women have had vaginal deliveries after a caesarean section. Ask your doctor what the reasons were for the last caesarean and whether they are likely to apply to the present baby.

Will the scar be very noticeable?
Doctors performing caesarean sections are very careful to make the incision just below the public hair-line and to keep it as small as they can. However, it has to be sufficiently large enough to allow the baby to be removed safely. Ask your doctor to show you where the cut will be and how long. It may take time for you to get used to the scar.

How long will it take to recover from a caesarean?
You may be in hospital for a week or longer. This will depend on how quickly you regain your health and how fit you are to cope with the demands of the baby.

Will the operation adversely affect my diabetic control?
No. Most caesareans are now performed under epidural anaesthetic. Good diabetic control can then be maintained throughout delivery. If a general anaesthetic is performed, doctors will carefully balance the diabetes so that the condition continues to be stable.

FERTILITY

Will I have difficulty conceiving?
A woman with diabetes is no less fertile than any other woman. However you may have problems if you are suffering from side effects of diabetes or have any other medical condition. Talk to your doctor.

Can I take fertility drugs?
Yes, if your doctor thinks these are necessary.

Can I have *in vitro* fertilisation?
Yes, if you are considered suitable for this form of treatment. However, you may have to go on a long waiting list.

OTHER QUESTIONS

Will pregnancy make my diabetes worse?
If you are already taking insulin, then your insulin doses will increase considerably during your pregnancy. However, this does not mean your condition has worsened. You should revert to your pre-pregnancy levels once the baby is born.

If you had diabetes that didn't need insulin before pregnancy, you will probably be put on insulin during your pregnancy so that optimum control can be reached. If you develop diabetes during pregnancy you will also be given insulin to take.

Will I be strapped to insulin and glucose drips throughout labour?
This is the traditional method of maintaining good diabetic control throughout labour. However, I did not have the drips and under epidural my blood glucose did not suffer.

Will the diabetes affect the production or quantity of breastmilk?
No. You should be able to feed with a slight adjustment to carbohydrate intake – usually about five extra portions.

GLOSSARY

acetone   A sweet smelling ketone that may be smelt on the breath if there are ketones in the blood.
acidosis   A build up of acids, usually ketones, in the blood.
adrenalin (epinephrine)   The hormone released from the central portion of the adrenal glands in response to a stress or emergency, e.g. an illness, a hypoglycaemic reaction, a fright.
albumen   A blood protein, which may appear in the urine when the kidneys are damaged.
amniocentesis   An operation to remove a small quantity of amniotic fluid which is used to test for fetal abnormalities.
anaesthesia (general)   Loss of sensation accompanied by loss of consciousness.
anaesthesia (local)   Loss of sensation of a part of the body; administered by an injection.
angina   Chest pain caused by insufficient blood supply to the heart muscle.
ankle oedema   Swelling of the ankles.
antenatal   The time during pregnancy prior to delivery.
antibodies   Special substances made by the body to protect it from specific disease or infection.
aorta   The largest artery in the body which carries blood from the heart through the chest and abdomen for distribution into other arteries.
artery   Vessel which carries blood from the heart to other parts of the body.
atherosclerosis   Hardening and furring up of the arteries.
autonomic nervous system   Nerves controlling largely automatic body functions such as heart beat, blood pressure and bowel movement.

autonomic neuropathy Abnormality of the nerves.
background retinopathy The common form of diabetic retinopathy with micro-aneurysms, dot and blot haemorrhages and exudates.
beta blocker Drugs which reduce high blood pressure, steady the heart and prevent angina.
beta cells The cells of the islets of Langerhans in the pancreas that produce insulin.
blood pressure (BP) Pressure at which blood circulates in the arteries.
Braxton Hicks contractions Painless uterine contractions which occur every 20 minutes throughout pregnancy.
breech presentation A baby presenting bottom first.
calorie A standard measurement of heat or energy used to assess the value of food. It is being replaced by the kilojoule. 1 Cal = 1,000 calories = 4.2 kilojoules.
carbohydrate (CHO) A class of foodstuff that is an important source of energy to the body. It is mainly represented by sugars and starches.
cardiac To do with the heart.
cataract An opacity of the lens of the eye that may be caused by long-standing diabetes.
catheter A tube used to drain urine out of the bladder.
cells The tiny building blocks from which the human body is made. Cell constituents are contained in a membrane.
cephalic presentation A baby presenting head first.
cervical canal The canal in the cervix from the uterus to the vagina.
cervix The lower part of the uterus.
chiropodist Someone who prevents and treats foot disorders.
cholesterol A fat which circulates in the blood and is obtained from animal fats in food and is a contributory factor in atherosclerosis.
chromosomes Rod-like structures, composed of genes. There are 23 pairs of chromosomes in each human cell (except the sex cells).
coma A state of unconsciousness. In diabetes this can result from hypoglycaemia or severe ketoacidosis.
conjunctivitis Inflammation of the conjunctiva (membrane covering the white of the eye and inner lid).
continuous subcutaneous insulin infusion (CSII) A system

for the constant pumping of insulin through a fine needle left under the skin all the time. Also known as an insulin pump.
coronary artery   Artery which supplies the heart muscle.
coronary thrombosis   Clot in an artery supplying heart muscle.
creatinine   Chemical produced by breakdown of protein in the body and passed through the kidneys into the urine. A measure of kidney function.
crowning   The moment of delivery of the baby's head.
cystitis   Inflammation of the urinary bladder.
dehydration   Being depleted of water. This occurs when the blood sugar is high for long periods, as in ketoacidosis.
dextrose   Simple sugar.
diabetes insipidus   Condition in which large volumes of insipid urine are passed. Caused by lack of anti-diuretic hormone.
diabetes mellitus   Condition in which the blood-glucose concentration is above normal, causing passage of large amounts (diabetes – a siphon) of sweet urine (mellitus – sweet like honey). Caused by inability of pancreas to produce sufficient insulin.
dialysis   Artificial filtration of fluid and waste products which are normally excreted in the urine by the kidneys.
diastolic blood pressure   Blood pressure between heart beats.
diet   What you eat.
dietitian   Someone who promotes a healthy diet and advises on dietary treatments.
diuretic   Pill which increases urinary fluid loss. Diuretics are used to treat cardiac failure and most are also effective blood-pressure lowering drugs.
dot and blot haemorrhage   Tiny bleeds into the retina in diabetic retinopathy.
dysmature   'Small for dates'. A baby that is smaller than would be expected for the duration of pregnancy.
dysuria   Pain or discomfort on passing urine.
echocardiography   Examination of heart using ultrasound waves from a probe run over skin of chest.
electrocardiogram (ECG or EKG)   Recording of electrical activity of heart muscle as it contracts and relaxes.
electrolytes   Blood chemicals sodium and potassium.
eneuresis   Involuntary passage of urine.

epidural anaesthetic An anaesthetic given by injection into an area of the back surrounding the spinal cord.
episiotomy Incision into the perineum to facilitate birth.
exchange diet One in which a fixed number of servings of carbohydrate, fat, protein and milk foods is prescribed so as to control total energy intake as well as the quantities of all major foodstuffs.
exudate Fatty deposit on the retina in retinopathy.
Fallopian tubes Tube connecting the ovary to the uterus.
fat Greasy or oily substance; fatty foods include butter, margarine, cheese, cooking oil, fried foods.
fatty acids These are the main components of body fat, in which they are combined with glycerol (glycerine).
femoral artery The main artery supplying each leg. The femoral pulse can be felt in the groin.
fetal distress A shortage of oxygen to the fetus.
fetus The baby while still in the womb.
fibre Roughage in food. Found in beans, lentils, peas, bran, wholemeal flour, potatoes, etc.
fructose A sugar found in fruit.
fundus The upper part of the uterus.
glaucoma Raised pressure inside the eye.
glucose A simple sugar obtained from carbohydrates in food. Glucose circulates in the bloodstream and is one of the body's main energy sources.
glucose tolerance The body's ability to process glucose.
glycaemia Glucose in the blood.
glycogen The form in which glucose is stored in the liver and muscles.
glycosuria Glucose in the urine.
glycosylated haemoglobin See haemoglobin HbA_1.
guar gum A substance which slows the absorption of carbohydrate from the gut.
haemoglobin HbA_1 Haemoglobin (oxygen-carrying chemical in red blood cells) to which glucose has become attached. A long-term measure of blood-glucose concentration.
haemorrhage Bleed.
hormone A chemical made in one part of the body and acting in another part of the body.
hyper- High, above normal.
hyperglycaemia High blood-glucose concentration (i.e. above normal).

hypertension High blood pressure.
hypo- Low, below normal.
hypoglycaemia Low blood-glucose concentration (i.e. below normal).
hypotension Low blood pressure.
hypothermia Low body temperature.
impotence Difficulty in obtaining or maintaining a penile erection.
insulin A hormone produced in cells of the islets of Langerhans in the pancreas. Essential for the entry of glucose into the body's cells.
insulin-dependent diabetes (IDD) See Type 1 diabetes.
insulin receptor Site on the cell surface where insulin acts.
intravenous glucose Glucose which is injected directly into a vein.
intravenous infusion Liquid such as water containing salt and glucose, which is slowly injected (usually out of a bottle and over a long period of time) directly into the bloodstream via a vein.
islet cells Cells which produce insulin.
islets of Langerhans Clusters of cells in the pancreas. One form of islet cells (beta cells) produces insulin.
juvenile-onset diabetes Diabetes starting in youth. This term implies a need for insulin treatment. Type I diabetes.
ketoacidis A state of severe insulin deficiency causing fat breakdown, ketone formation and acidification of the blood.
ketones Products of a breakdown of fat which smell of acetone or pear-drops and make the blood acid.
kilocalories, Cals or kcals A measure of energy, for example in food or used up in exercise.
kilojoules Another measure of energy. One kilocalorie = 4.2 kilojoules.
lactation The process of milk production.
lactose The sugar found in milk.
left ventricle Chamber of the heart which pumps oxygenated blood into the aorta.
lens The part of the eye responsible for focusing (like the lens of a camera).
lipid General name for fats found in the body.
liver Large organ in upper right abdomen which acts as an energy store, chemical factory and detoxifying unit, and which produces bile.

lochia Blood-stained discharge from the vagina after delivery.
maturity-onset diabetes Diabetes starting over the age of 30. This term usually implies that the person is not completely insulin deficient, at least initially. Non-insulin dependent diabetes. Type II diabetes.
meconium Thick dark substance present in the baby's rectum before and after birth.
metabolism Chemical processing of substances in the body.
microaneurysm Tiny blow-out in capillary wall in retina of eye.
micturition Passing urine.
millilitre (ml) A measure of volume of a liquid.
millimole per litre (mmol) A measure of the concentration of a substance.
multigravida A woman during her second or subsequent pregnancy.
neonatal death Death within 28 days of birth.
nerve Cable carrying signals to or from the brain via the spinal chord.
neuropathy Abnormality of the nerves.
nocturia Passing urine at night.
non-insulin-dependent diabetes (NIDD) Diabetes in which insulin treatment is not essential initially. See Type II diabetes.
obese Overweight, fat.
obesity Condition of being overweight or fat.
obstetrician A doctor who specialises in pregnancy.
oedema Swelling.
oestriol A hormone secreted by the placenta. Low levels may indicate fetal distress and an underweight baby as well as the chance of stillbirth.
ophthalmologist An eye specialist.
oral Taken by mouth.
ovulation The production of an egg or ovum from the ovary.
oxytocin A hormone which makes the uterus contract.
paediatrician A doctor who specialises in newborn babies and children.
palpitations Awareness of irregular or abnormally fast heart beat.
pancreas Abdominal gland producing digestive enzymes,

paraesthesia Pins and needles or tingling.
-pathy Disease, abnormality, e.g. neuropathy, retinopathy.
perineum The area between the anus and the vagina.
peripheral nervous system Nerves supplying the muscles attached to the skeleton and registering body sensation such as touch, pain, temperature.
photocoagulation Light treatment of retinopathy.
placenta The afterbirth. It transfers nutrients from the mother to the baby in the womb as well as waste products from the baby to the mother.
polydipsia Drinking large volumes of fluid.
polyunsaturated fats Fats containing vegetable oils such as sunflower seed oil.
polyuria Passing large volumes of urine frequently.
postnatal After delivery.
pre-eclampsia A condition sometimes found in pregnancy, characterised by raised blood pressure, swollen ankles and fingers, and protein in the urine.
primigravida A woman having her first pregnancy.
protein Dietary constituent required for body growth and repair.
proteinuria Protein in the urine.
pruritus vulvae Itching of the vulva or perineum.
pyelonephritis Kidney infection.
receptor Site on the cell wall with which a chemical or hormone links.
renal To do with the kidney.
renal glycosuria The presence of glucose in the urine because of an abnormally low renal threshold for glucose.
renal threshold Blood glucose concentration above which glucose overflows into the urine.
retina Light sensitive tissue at the back of the eye.
retinopathy Abnormality of the retina.
rhesus disease The damage or destruction of the red blood cells of a rhesus positive baby.
risk factor A factor which makes you more likely to develop a particular problem than someone who does not have this factor.
saturated fats Animal fats, e.g. in dairy products, meat.
stillbirth The birth of a dead baby after 28 weeks of pregnancy.
stroke Abnormality of brain function (e.g. weakness of arm

or leg) due to disease of the arteries supplying oxygen to the brain or damage to the brain.
subcutaneous Under the skin.
subcutaneous fat The fatty tissues under the skin.
systolic blood pressure Pumping pressure of the heart, as measured in the arteries.
testosterone Male sex hormone.
thrombosis Clotting of blood.
thrush Candidiasis or moniliasis. Fungal infection caused by *Candida albicans* fungus. Produces white creamy patches and intense itching and soreness.
trimester One third of pregnancy. First trimester 1–14 weeks, second trimester 14–28 weeks, third trimester 28 weeks to term.
Type I diabetes Diabetes due to complete insulin deficiency for which treatment with insulin is essential. Lack of insulin leads to rapid illness and ketone production. Juvenile-onset diabetes, insulin-dependent diabetes.
Type II diabetes Diabetes due to inefficiency of insulin action or relative insulin deficiency, which can usually be managed without insulin injections, at least initially. Ketone formation is less likely. Maturity-onset diabetes, non-insulin-dependent diabetes.
ulcer Open sore.
ultrasound scan Scan of part of the body using sound waves.
urea Blood chemical; waste substance excreted in urine.
ureter Tube from the kidney to the urinary bladder.
urethra Tube from the urinary bladder to the outside.
urinary incontinence Unintentional leakage of urine.
urinary retention Retention of urine in the bladder because it cannot be passed.
urinary tract infection (UTI) Infection of urine drainage system.
uterus Womb.
visual acuity Sharpness of vision.
vulva The external part of the female reproductive organs.

USEFUL ADDRESSES AND TELEPHONE NUMBERS

UK

Abortion Anonymous
01-350 2229

ASH – Action on Smoking and Health
5–11 Mortimer Street
London W1N 7RH
01-637 9843
Information on hazards of smoking and advice on how to give up.

Association for the Advancement of Maternity Care
Sycamores
Chilbolton
Stockbridge
Hampshire

AIMS – Association for Improvements in the Maternity Services
163 Liverpool Road
London N1 0RF
01-278 5628

Association for Post-Natal Illness
7 Gowan Avenue
Fulham
London SW6 6RH

Association of Breast Feeding Mothers
131 Maylow Road
London SE26
01-778 4769

Association of Radical Midwives
8A The Drive
London SW20 8TG

British Diabetic Association
10 Queen Anne Street
London W1M 0BD
01-323 1531

British Heart Foundation
01-935 0185 during office hours

British Right to a Child Trust
Skye House
Holmfirth
West Yorkshire HD7 1RU
048 489 3386

Brook Advisory Centre
153a East Street
London SE17 2SD
01-708 1234/1390
Brook Advisory Centres can be found all over the country. Check your telephone book for your nearest centre.

Caesarean Support Network
11 Duke Street
Astley
Manchster M29 7BG
0942 878076

Care
790 Crookson Road
Glasgow G35 7TT
041-882 6080
The Scottish Association for Care and Support after Termination for Abnormality.

Compassionate Friends
6 Denmark Street
Bristol BS1 5DQ
0272 292778
Self-help group for people who have lost their children.

CRUSE
Cruse House
126 Sheen Road
Richmond
Surrey
01-940 4818
Counselling service for the bereaved.

CRY-SIS
London WC1N 3XX
01-404 5011
For parents of babies who cry a lot.

Diabetic Pregnancy Network
Diabetes Care Department
British Diabetic Association
10 Queen Anne Street
London W1M 0BD
01-323 1531

Family Planning Association
27–35 Mortimer Street
London W1N 7RJ
01-636 7866

Family Network
National Childrens' Home
85 Highbury Park
London N5 1UD
01-226 2033
Phone-in service to help parents in any way possible.

FORESIGHT
The Old Vicarage
Church Lane
Whitley

Godalming
Surrey GU8 5PN
042879 4500
Pre-conceptual care. Offers a wide range of booklets including *Guidelines for Future Parents*, £2 plus SAE.

Foresight Vitamin Service
Mrs P. Aschwarden
Dellrose Cottage
Littlewick Road
Lower Knaphill
Woking
Surrey GU21 2JU
Will supply Foresight mineral and vitamin supplements.

Healthcall
Main number 0898 600600
24 hours

Healthline
01-980 4848
2–10 pm

Health Education Authority
78 New Oxford Street
London WC1A 1AH
01-631 0930

Impotence Information Centre
Freepost
158–162 High Street
Staines
TW18 1BR

La Leche League
BM 3424
London WC1V 6XX
01-242 1278

Marie Stopes House
108 Whitfield Street
London W1P 6BE
01-388 2585/0662

Marie Stopes Centre
10 Queen Square
Leeds LS2 8AJ
0532 440685

Marie Stopes Centre
1 Police Street
Manchester M2 7LQ
061-832 4260

Maternity Alliance
15 Britannia Street
London WC1X 9JP
01-837 1265
Information on legal rights and benefits.

Medical Advisory Service
01-994 9874
24 hours

MENCAP – Royal Society for Mentally Handicapped Children and Adults
117–123 Golden Lane
London EC1Y 0RT
01-253 9433

Miscarriage Association
18 Stoney Brook Close
West Bretton
Wakefield
West Yorkshire WF4 4TP
0924 85515

National Association for the Childless
318 Summer Lane
Birmingham B19 3PL
021-359 4887/2113

National Association of Ovulation Method Instructors
47 Heathhurst Road
Sanderstead
South Croydon
Surrey CR2 0BB

National Childbirth Trust
9 Queensborough Terrace
Bayswater
London W2 3TB
01-221 3833

National Council for One Parent Families
255 Kentish Town Road
London NW5 2LX
01-267 1361

NIPPERS
Perinatal Research Unit
St Mary's Hospital
Praed Street
London W2 1NY
01-262 1280
Premature babies.

OPUS – National Organisation for Parents Under Stress
106 Godstone Road
Whyteleafe
Surrey CR3 0EB
01-643 0469

The Patients' Association
Room 33, 18 Charing Cross Road
London WC2
01-240 0671

PETS – Pre-Eclamptic Toxaemia Society
33 Keswick Avenue
Hullbridge
Essex SS5 6JL
0702 231689

Pregnancy Advisory Service
Austy Manor
Wootton, Wawen
West Midlands B95 6BX
05642 3225

Relaxation for Living
29 Burwood Park Road
Walton-on-Thames
Surrey KY12 5LH
0932 227826
Supply relaxation tapes and cassettes.

SAFTA – Support after Termination for Abnormalities
22 Upper Woburn Place
London WC1 0EP
01-388 1382

Society to Support Home Confinements
Margaret Whyte
17 Laburnam Avenue
Durham City DH1 4HA

Stillbirth and Neonatal Death Society
29–31 Euston Road
London NW1 2SD
01-833 2851/2

TAMBA – Twins and Multiple Births Association
292 Valley Road
Lillington
Leamington Spa, CV32 7UE

Ulster Pregnancy Advisory Association
719a Lisburn Road
Belfast 9
0232 381345

Voluntary Council for Handicapped Children
8 Wakley Street
London EC1 7QE

Women's Reproductive Rights Information Centre
52–4 Featherstone Street
London EC1Y 8RT
01-251 6332

Working Mothers Association
23 Webbs Road
London SW11 6RU
01-228 3757

AUSTRALIA

Australian Federation of FPAs
Suite 603, Roden Cutler House
24 Campbell Street
Sydney, NSW 2000

Diabetes Education and Assessment Centre
74 Herbert Street
St Leonards, NSW 2065
(02) 433476; 4384584

Diabetes Foundation (Vic)
100 Collins Street
Melbourne, Vic 3000
(03) 638793

Diabetes Research Foundation of WA
Queen Elizabeth II Medical Centre
Hollywood
Perth, WA 6000
381 3329

Diabetic Association
86 Hampden Road
Bay Point
Hobart, Tas. 7000
(002) 345223

Diabetic Association
19 Irwin Street
Perth, WA 6091
325 7174; 325 9368

Diabetic Association of NSW
250 Pitt Street
Sydney, NSW 2000
(02) 264 6851; 264 6909

Diabetic Association of Queensland
Ann Street
Brisbane, Qld 4000
(07) 229 1986

Diabetic Association of SA
Eleanor Harrald Building
Frome Road
Adelaide, SA 5000
(08) 223 7848

Diabetic Information Centre
Woden Valley Hospital
Yamba Drive
Garran, ACT 2605
(062) 810433

CANADA

The Canadian Diabetes Association
78 Bond Street
Toronto, Ontario M5B 2J8

EIRE

Irish Family Planning Clinic
Cathal Brugha Street Clinic
Dublin 1
Dublin 727276/727363
Similar service to the FPA within the confines of Irish law.

NEW ZEALAND

The New Zealand FPA Inc.
PO Box 68200
214 Karangahape
Newton, Auckland

UNITED STATES

The American Diabetes Association
National Service Center
1660 Duke Street
Alexandria, VA 22314

National Diabetes Information Clearing House
Box NDIC
Bethesda, MD 20205

Planned Parenthood Federation of America
Head office:
2010 Massachusetts Avenue, NW, Suite 500
Washington DC 20036
(202) 785 3351

Northern region:
2625 Butterfield Road
Oak Brook, Illinois 60521
(312) 986 9270

Southern region:
3030 Peachtree Road, NW, Room 303
Atlanta, Georgia 30305

Western region:
333 Broadway, 3rd Floor
San Francisco, California 94133
(415) 956 8856

INDEX

Page numbers in *italic* refer to the illustrations.

abnormalities, 4, 7, 13, 120; and breastfeeding, 110
abortion, 57, 142
AFP (Alphafetoprotein), 2, 23
AIDS, 71
alcohol, 3, 15
amniocentesis, 10, 22
amniotic fluid, 33; analysis, 25
anaemia, 30
antenatal: care, 19–34; clinic, 22–30
arteries, hardening, 59
Asian women, 56
aspirin, 57

baby, 116–124
baby blues, 101
Balance magazine, vii
barrier methods, contraception, 139–40
Billings contraceptive method, 141
bladder, 28
bleeding, 33, 34
blood glucose, 1, 2, 3, 27, 30; effects of, 13; profile, *36*; and sex, 136
blood-glucose tests, 21, 35; equipment, 83; extra injections, 4; home measurements, 35, 39; monitoring meters, 37, 38
blood pressure, 10, 13; oedema, 26
blood sugar *see* blood glucose
blood tests: anaemia, 30; levels, 14
breastfeeding, 102–115, 144; by demand, 110; discontinuing, 111;
how to, 103, *103*, *104*; problems, 109
breastmilk, 105, 146
breast, 28
breathing difficulties, 120
Brewer, Gail Sforza, 26
Brewer, Dr Tom, 26
British Diabetic Association, vii; Care Dept, 129; pregnancy pack, vii

caesareans, vii, 2, 4, 13, 94–7, 145; and breastfeeding, 107; and epidurals, 97, *97*
caffeine, 57
calcium, 80, 119
calories, 16
carbohydrates, 77, 79
case-studies: breastfeeding, 111–115; caesareans, 95–6; gestational diabetes, 52–6; hypoglycaemia, 44; labour, 95–7; miscarriage, 32–3; pre-conception, 9–12; pregnancy and diabetes, 1–5; stillbirth, 121–3
cataracts, 58
childbirth, 83–100
coil, contraceptive, 138
coitus interruptus, 141
colostrum, 103
coma, 26
conception: diabetic control, 7; diet, 17, 18; maternal age, 14, 15
condoms, 139
congenital abnormalities, 4, 7, 13, 120

contraception, 6, 31, 136–42, *137*; calendar method, 141; coil, 138; injections, 140; mucus method, 141; pill, 137; temperature method, 141
convulsions, 26
cycling, 64

Davis, Adelle, 17
demand feeding, 110
depression, 3, 31
diabetes: coping with baby, 130; during labour, 88; gestational, 51, 56; pregnancy, 146; research, 81
diabetic antenatal clinics, 1
diabetic clinics, 4
diabetic physician, vii, 6
Diabetic Pregnancy Network, 19, 20, 157
diabetic retinopathy, 6, 58
diaphragm, contraceptive, 139
diet, 1, 5, 16, 27, 59, 76–82; breastfeeding, 105; and conception, 17
dietitian, 6
Directory of Private Hospitals & Health Services, 21
drinking, 3, 15
Driver and Vehicle Licensing Centre, 58
Dunn Clinical Research Centre, 61, 72

ECG (electrocardiogram), 6, 8, epidurals, 2, 89; and caesareans, 97
episiotomy, 31, 92, *92*
exercise, 16, 59, 62–5
exercises, *66–70*, 68–70
eyes: glaucoma, 58; retinopathy, 6, 58

false labour, 87
fats, 80
feet: gangrene, 59; problems, 59, 60, 83; symptoms of problems, 60
fertility, 145
fetal monitoring, 90–2, *91*

fetal movement, 28, 30, 50; absence of, 34, 123
folic acid, 15, 80
Fuller, Nigel J., 72
fungal infections, thrush, 49

genetic counselling, 11
German measles, 7, 15
gestational diabetes, 51–6; symptoms, 51
glaucoma, 58
glossary, 147–54
glucagon, *45*, 46
glucocheck meters, 1
glucose: hypoglycaemia, 5; hypoglycaemia detection, 35; tablets, 45, 83; test strips, 3
glycaemic index, 76
glycosylated haemoglobin *see* HbA1
growth of fetus, 75

haemorrhoids, 31
HbA1, 7, 8, 13
HbA1 test, 37
health visitor, 126
heart disease, 14
heredity, 117
home births, 100
hormone drips, 2
hormone tests, 30
hospital, 144; private, 21; questions to ask, 20
housework, 127
HPL, (human placental lactogen), 25
hunger, 61, 106
hydramnios, 99
hyperglycaemia, 47, 48
hypocalcaemia, babies, 119
hypoglycaemia, 5, 7, 9, 13; coma, 4; detection of, 35; drunkeness, 15; symptoms, 42, 48; treatment, 45
Hypostop, 46, *47*

immunisation, 7, 15
incontinence, stress, 31
induction, vii, 13, 84; advantages 85; disadvantages, 85; methods, 85

infections, 49, 101
infertility, 17, 145
injecting, in front of children, 130
Insulatard, 1
insulin: clear, 39; cloudy, 39; dosage, 10; infusion pumps, 41, *41*; insulin/glucose drips, 2; pens, 5, 39, 40, *40*
intercourse, 133–6
intercourse, recommended positions during pregnancy, 134
inter-uterine contraceptive device (IUCD or coil), 138
iron, 80

jaundice, 2, 120
jogging, 64

keep-fit, 65
ketones, 2, 25, 50
kidneys, 6, 26, 58
King's College Hospital, 19
Kitzinger, Sheila, 133

labour, 18, 83–101, *89*; false, 87; length, 88; premature, 33; stages, 88
Let Us Have Healthy Children, 17
lungs, 13

macrosomia, 13, 75, 76, 120
Masters and Johnson, 135
mastitis, 109
mealtimes, 128
Medic-Alert bracelet, *48*
Medic-Alert disc, 58
Medical Market Information Ltd, 21
Medical Research Council, Dunn Nutrition Centre, 61, 72
midwife, 125
miscarriage, 31, 32, 33
Mixtard, 1
morning sickness, 27
morning-after pill, 140
mucus method, contraception, 141

National Childbirth Trust, 19, 129, 160
natural childbirth, 98

nightfeeding, 110
nutrition, 72–82

obstetrician, 6
oedema, 10
Oestriol, 25
oestrogen pill, 140
oils, 80
organisation, 126
oxytocin, 86

pain, 31, 32
pessaries, 85
pill, contraceptive, 137
placenta, 74, 75
postnatal: check up, 31; depression, 101, 129; infections, 101
pre-conception, 6–18; counselling, 4, 8, 12
pre-conceptual care, 9
pre-eclampsia, 13, 26, 99
pregnancy pack, vii
pregnancy tests, 7, 7
premature baby, 107
private hospitals, 21
protein, 2, 17, 79

relaxation, 67
renal: disease, 14; threshold, 26
respiratory distress, 13
retinopathy, 6, 14, 58
risks, to baby, 12
rubella, 7, 15
rupture of membranes, 86

sex, 133–6
shopping, 127
sleeping, 29, 127
smoking, 3, 14, 59
snacks, 62
special care unit, *118*, *119*, 143
sponge, contraceptive, 140
Steele, Dr Judith, 6, 121
sterilisation, 141
stillbirth, 4, 121–3; grief, 124
stress incontinence, 31
stretch marks, 28
sweeteners, 78, 80
swimming, 63

telemetry, 38
thrush, 49
thyroxine, 57
toxaemia, 2, 26
transitional milk, 103
twins, 121, 143; breastfeeding, 108, *108*

ultrasound, 23, 24, 27–30
urine test strips, 25

varicose veins, 31
vegetarian diet, 81
Velosulin, 1
vitamins, 5, 17

walking, 63
weight, 51, 52; birth, 11, 12; gain, 60, 74; loss, 6, 7
What Every Pregnant Woman Should Know, 26